BEATING MIGRAINES

7 Natural Secrets for Lasting Relief

Dr. Joseph Jacobs, DPT, ACN

Second Edition, January 2026

Published by ASTR Institute
614 E HWY 50 #169, Clermont, FL 34711

ASTR

ASTRinstitute.com

Disclaimer

This book, authored by Dr. Joseph Jacobs and published by the ASTR Institute, is intended for informational purposes only and presents medical research findings. It is not a substitute for professional medical advice, diagnosis, or treatment. Dr. Joseph Jacobs, the ASTR Institute, and its affiliates do not endorse or assume responsibility for any specific medical treatments or procedures discussed in this book. We strongly advise readers to consult with their healthcare providers regarding the applicability of any aspects of the content to their own health and well-being.

The statements contained herein have not been evaluated by the Food and Drug Administration. The products mentioned are not designed to diagnose, cure, treat, or prevent any disease. Individual results may vary, and we cannot guarantee that you will achieve the same outcomes as those detailed in our case studies, testimonials, and treatment videos. Success varies per individual, and one person's results do not guarantee similar outcomes for another.

If you have medical concerns, consult with your healthcare provider, physician, or another qualified medical professional. Dr. Joseph Jacobs, the ASTR Institute, and their associated organizations and individuals disclaim any liability for actions, services, or products acquired through this book, our videos, website, or any of our media channels.

Table of Contents

Online Resources

How to Access Online Resources

Throughout this book, you'll find barcodes that link to additional online resources. Here's how to use them:

1. Open the camera app on your smartphone.
2. Point the camera at the barcode.
3. A notification will appear with a link. Tap the notification to open the link in your browser.

Triumph Over Trials: My Journey from Disability to Victory

After my second cancer treatment, I was suffering from chronic fatigue, migraines, muscle and joint pain. I reached out to at least seven doctors, but I could not find relief. Unfortunately, they had two responses. First, they said my blood labs looked normal. I learned from my studies in nutrition that this happened because they did not order the correct labs to figure out the root cause of my issues. The second response was that I was a hopeless case. This made me realize that if I wanted to overcome my disability, I had to look for a solution on my own. It was a difficult time in my life. Due to my pain and fatigue, it used to take me 10 minutes just to walk from the living room to the bathroom, about 20 feet away. I was very depressed and angry because, at 30 years old, I was facing numerous health issues and had a poor quality of life without any answers.

I spent countless hours and years studying nutrition, psychology, behavioral modification, anatomy, physiology, ergonomics, and other medical topics in hopes of finding an answer. At the same time, I was frustrated that the techniques I learned in medical school only provided short-term results with no lasting relief. I tried what I learned in school, such as stretching, exercises, electrical stimulation, various massage techniques, manual therapy, joint mobilization, and myofascial release, but nothing provided long-term results. So, I started to look at medical studies to guide me through this process. After reviewing over 16,000 medical research papers with assistance from medical students, I was shocked and disappointed by the results. Based on these studies, the following treatments either provided no pain reduction or only short-term pain reduction:

- NSAIDs
- Opioids
- Cortisone shots
- Exercises
- Stretching
- Massage
- Joint mobilization or manipulation
- Acupuncture
- Dry needling
- Instrument-assisted soft tissue mobilization

I have dedicated my life to researching all current traditional medical approaches to treating pain. I've found that the majority of these approaches primarily focus on relieving symptoms rather than addressing the root cause of the pain. The techniques I learned in school, still used in today's modern medical world, have their origins in ancient healing practices such as manipulation, massage, stretching, and exercise. These methods were used by the Romans, Greeks, and Egyptians to increase flexibility, strengthen muscles, and alleviate pain. Today's medicine has added treatments like cold, heat, electrical stimulation, and joint adjustment to this list. However, overwhelming evidence from published medical studies shows no promising long-term relief from any of these methods.

For instance, one systematic review conducted by the University of Ottawa, Canada, which reviewed 270 research studies, concluded that the benefits of massage, acupuncture, and spine adjustment treatments were mostly evident immediately or shortly after treatment, then faded over time. With compelling data like this, it is perplexing how we continue to treat patients with modalities that do not effectively address their long-term needs. Instead of focusing so much on the body's symptoms, we need to start questioning why these symptoms are present in the first place and why they keep returning.

This question guided me through an intense investigative research process over five years. From this research, I concluded that there are seven aspects of chronic pain that, when treated simultaneously, can lead to long-term pain relief. In my book, **Pain No More**, I outline seven key elements that must be addressed simultaneously to effectively relieve chronic pain. I also found that the BioPsychosocial model is an effective treatment approach for long-term pain reduction. So, I studied the BioPsychosocial model in depth and realized that my medical education was lacking in nutrition knowledge. I spent thousands of hours reading and studying nutrition and bought any book that I felt could help me understand the body better.

During this time, my wife had chronic jaw pain due to stress at work. I tried everything I learned from school on her, but nothing provided long-term pain relief. One day she woke up with lockjaw, unable to speak or open her mouth. She asked me to try anything. I told her that I had tried everything I knew, but nothing worked. So, I reached inside her mouth and experimented with several maneuvers. After a few minutes, she was able to open her mouth and was pain-free. I was dumbfounded and had no idea what had just happened. It took me several days to understand the physiology of the maneuvers I had performed. I then started experimenting with the same concept, applying it to the whole body to relieve both my pain and my patients' pain.

After several months of using my hands to implement the new maneuvers I had come up with, I realized I could not do that long-term. My hands were very sore, and I suffered from pain every night. I told my wife that this was not sustainable because I was in so much pain from using my hands. While patients were getting relief, I was suffering. My wife suggested that I use tools instead of my hands. So, I went to a hardware store and bought rubber, plastic, and metal to cut and design tools and devices to replace my hand maneuvers. Thankfully, this provided even faster results for my patients without me feeling soreness from working on them.

I was able to overcome my chronic fatigue and migraines by running comprehensive lab tests. These tests revealed several vitamin, mineral, and hormonal imbalances. Additionally, I overcame my chronic joint and muscle pain through the biopsychosocial (BPS) model and the tools and devices I invented. I also reinvented the biopsychosocial model to be implemented by a single healthcare provider and called it ASTR treatment.

My journey toward developing the ASTR diet was driven by personal challenges and professional insights. I experienced significant frustration with various diets that often left me feeling fatigued and unsatisfied. Through an extensive review of research studies, I also uncovered potential health risks associated with extreme dietary approaches. These experiences inspired me to create the ASTR Diet as a healthier, evidence-based alternative, which I share in my book **Eat to Heal**.

For years, I suffered from debilitating migraines, searching for lasting relief beyond temporary fixes. My journey as both a patient and a healthcare provider led me to dedicate 15 years to researching, studying, and testing effective solutions. Through this process, I developed a comprehensive approach that transformed my own health and has helped countless patients overcome chronic migraines. In this book, I share these evidence-based strategies, solutions that I have refined through experience and clinical practice. My hope is that this book serves as a practical guide to empower you on your path to recovery, providing the tools and knowledge needed to reclaim a pain-free life.

The Roadmap to Healing

The Roadmap to Healing: A Comprehensive Approach to Beating Migraines

Migraines are one of the most complex and misunderstood conditions, often presenting as more than just severe headaches. They are a systemic issue, influenced by multiple underlying factors that can vary from person to person. Through 15 years of research, clinical practice, and personal experience, I have found that migraines are rarely triggered by a single element. Instead, they are the result of a combination of factors, such as food sensitivities, medications, chronic stress, hormonal imbalances, environmental toxins, and deficiencies in essential vitamins and minerals. It is common to find that migraine sufferers have at least five to seven contributing triggers, making an individualized and holistic approach to treatment essential for lasting relief.

In this chapter, I introduce a structured roadmap to healing, seven natural secrets to lasting relief, designed to address the root causes of migraines rather than just suppressing symptoms. These elements are interconnected, and for the best results, it is crucial to implement all seven. Each component plays a key role in restoring balance to the body, reducing inflammation, and optimizing the nervous and vascular systems. When one or more of these factors are overlooked, migraines often persist or return, which is why a comprehensive approach is necessary.

By following this roadmap, you are not just managing your migraines; you are taking control of your health and actively working toward eliminating them at their source. **This method is not about quick fixes or temporary relief but about equipping your body with the tools it needs to heal naturally and sustainably.** Just as I did for my own migraines and as my patients have done, through dedication and consistency, you can break free from the cycle of chronic migraines and regain your quality of life.

Case Studies

This chapter presents real-life case studies of individuals who have successfully implemented the ASTR approach to overcome chronic migraines. Each case study highlights the patient's unique challenges, treatment strategies, and outcomes. These stories provide valuable insights and inspiration for readers, demonstrating the effectiveness of a holistic, science-based approach to migraine relief.

Understanding Migraines

This chapter provides a comprehensive exploration of migraines, including their neurological and physiological mechanisms. It delves into the role of the trigeminovascular system, cortical spreading depression, neurotransmitter imbalances, and genetic predispositions. Readers will gain a deeper understanding of how migraines develop, the various types of migraines, and the factors that contribute to their frequency and severity. This chapter lays the foundation for the holistic approach to migraine relief presented in the book.

Navigating the Healing Journey: How Your Body Recovers Naturally

This chapter will explore the normal body healing cycle, detailing the intricate processes that allow the body to repair and recover naturally. It will explain how the body's immune system, nervous system, and cellular mechanisms work together to promote healing, reduce inflammation, and restore balance. In contrast, the chapter will also examine the chronic migraine cycle, highlighting the internal disruptions that prevent proper healing. Chronic migraines often result from a combination of neurovascular dysfunction, heightened pain sensitivity, inflammation, and metabolic imbalances, leading to recurring and persistent pain. By understanding the differences between the body's natural healing response and the migraine cycle, readers will gain valuable insights into how to break free from the repetitive nature of chronic migraines and support their body's ability to heal effectively.

7 Natural Secrets

1. Migraine-Triggering Foods

Certain foods can contribute to migraine attacks by triggering inflammatory responses, disrupting neurotransmitter function, or affecting vascular stability. This chapter outlines the most common migraine-triggering foods, including processed sugars, artificial additives, and histamine-rich foods. It introduces the

ASTR Diet's elimination approach to help readers identify their personal triggers and transition to a migraine-friendly, nutrient-dense diet.

2. Imbalance: Vitamins, Minerals, and Hormones

Nutritional deficiencies and hormonal imbalances play a critical role in migraine frequency and severity. This chapter discusses how deficiencies in magnesium, vitamin D, B vitamins, and other essential nutrients contribute to migraines. It also explores how hormonal fluctuations, particularly estrogen, cortisol, and thyroid hormones, affect migraine patterns. Practical strategies for restoring balance through diet, supplementation, and lifestyle modifications are provided.

3. Posture

Poor posture, especially in the cervical spine, is a significant but often overlooked contributor to migraines. This chapter examines how misalignments in the neck and shoulders can lead to muscle tension, nerve compression, and reduced blood flow to the brain. Readers will learn about postural correction techniques, ergonomic adjustments, and exercises that can alleviate migraine symptoms and prevent recurrence.

4. Stress Management

Chronic stress is a major migraine trigger, as it leads to hormonal imbalances, muscle tension, and heightened nervous system sensitivity. This chapter introduces effective stress management techniques, including mindfulness, deep breathing exercises, and relaxation strategies. It also discusses how emotional health and unresolved trauma can impact migraine frequency and provides practical steps for fostering mental and emotional resilience.

5. Fibrotic Tissue

Scar tissue and fibrotic adhesions can develop in response to injuries, chronic inflammation, or repetitive strain, leading to muscle tightness and restricted movement. This chapter explores how fibrotic tissue in the neck and shoulders can contribute to migraines by impairing circulation and nerve function.

6. Fascial Restriction

The fascia, a connective tissue network that surrounds muscles and organs, plays a crucial role in movement and pain regulation. When the fascia becomes restricted, it can lead to tension and discomfort, including migraine-related pain. This chapter explains the connection between fascial restrictions and migraines and introduces methods for restoring fascial health.

7. Behavior Modification

Long-term migraine relief requires lasting changes in lifestyle habits and behaviors. This chapter examines the impact of sleep patterns, hydration, physical activity, and environmental factors on migraine prevention. It provides guidance on habit formation, self-monitoring techniques, and strategies for sustaining positive lifestyle changes to ensure lasting migraine relief.

Conclusion

The final chapter summarizes the key takeaways from the book and reinforces the importance of a comprehensive, natural approach to migraine management. It encourages readers to take an active role in their healing journey, emphasizing the power of lifestyle changes, nutritional support, and targeted therapies. The chapter concludes with actionable steps for implementing the ASTR approach and achieving lasting relief from migraines.

Case Studies & Research

All case studies presented in this book illustrate that a holistic approach to migraine treatment can be effectively implemented by a single healthcare provider. A holistic approach considers the interconnected systems of the body, addressing not only the symptoms of migraines but also the underlying causes that contribute to their recurrence. This method integrates multiple elements, including nutritional balance, musculoskeletal health, stress management, lifestyle adjustments, and behavioral modifications, to create a comprehensive treatment plan tailored to the individual's needs.

By focusing on the root causes rather than just symptom management, a holistic approach can identify and correct deficiencies in vitamins, minerals, and hormones. It also addresses postural imbalances, reduces fibrotic tissue and fascial restrictions, and implements behavior modification techniques to support long-term healing. This integrative method not only helps in alleviating pain but also promotes long-term wellness and prevention of future migraine episodes.

The case studies and recorded live treatment videos available online provide real-life examples of how this approach is applied in practice. These materials demonstrate the step-by-step process of evaluating and treating migraines holistically, offering insight into how a healthcare provider can systematically assess and address each contributing factor. To watch these case studies and treatment videos, use the barcode provided in this book or visit the following link:

https://advancedsofttissuerelease.com/treatment-videos-2/

Case Studies & Research

Case Study 1: **10 Years of Migraines, Daily Headaches, and Jaw Pain**
Diagnosis: Migraines and jaw pain.
Symptoms: Migraines; jaw, ear, temporal, face, and neck pain; constant daily headaches at 4/10 that increase throughout the day; teeth grinding.
Previous Failed Treatments: Dentist, neurologist, medication, migraine medications, massage therapy, chiropractor, acupuncture, and essential oils.
Length of Injury: 10 years.
Pain Level on a Scale of 0 to 10: 4-8/10.
Treatment: Treatment included releasing fibrotic tissue, addressing fascia restrictions, decreasing inflammation, improving ergonomics, and implementing an anti-inflammatory diet.
Outcome: Symptoms resolved.

Case Study 2: **4 Months of Migraines, Neck and Shoulder Pain**
Diagnosis: Migraines & neck and shoulder Pain.
Symptoms: Migraines several times a week, neck and shoulder soreness, fatigue, sensitivity to light, nausea, migraine aura, and eye pressure.
Previous Failed Treatments: Medication and migraine medications.
Length of Injury: 4 months.
Pain Level on a Scale of 0 to 10: 4-5/10.
Treatment: Treatment included releasing fibrotic tissue, addressing fascia restrictions, decreasing inflammation, improving ergonomics, and implementing an anti-inflammatory diet.
Outcome: Symptoms resolved.

Case Study 3: **5 Years of Daily Tension Headaches, Neck, and Jaw Pain**
Diagnosis: Daily tension headaches.
Symptoms: Daily headaches, blurry vision, jaw pain, neck pain, jaw clicks, and throbbing head pain.
Previous Failed Treatments: Neurologist, ENT doctor, various physical therapists, chiropractor, neck specialist, botox shots, cortisone shots, muscle relaxers, and medication.
Length of Injury: 5 years.
Pain Level on a Scale of 0 to 10: 4-5/10.
Treatment: Treatment included releasing fibrotic tissue, addressing fascia restrictions, decreasing inflammation, improving ergonomics, and implementing

an anti-inflammatory diet.
Outcome: Symptoms resolved.

Case Study 4: **2 Years of Tension Headaches**
Diagnosis: Tension headaches.
Symptoms: Almost daily headaches and neck stiffness.
Previous Failed Treatments: medication.
Length of Injury: 2 years
Pain Level on a Scale of 0 to 10: 4-6/10.
Treatment: Treatment included releasing fibrotic tissue, addressing fascia restrictions, decreasing inflammation, improving ergonomics, and implementing an anti-inflammatory diet.
Outcome: Symptoms resolved.

Case Study 5: **Locked Jaw and Migraines**
Diagnosis: Locked jaw and migraines.
Symptoms: Locked jaw, migraines, face and neck pain, inability to chew, and inability to sleep.
Previous Failed Treatments: Dentist and medication.
Length of Injury: 1 week.
Pain Level on a Scale of 0 to 10: 9-10/10.
Treatment: Treatment included releasing fibrotic tissue, addressing fascia restrictions, decreasing inflammation, improving ergonomics, and implementing an anti-inflammatory diet.
Outcome: Symptoms resolved.

Case Study 6: **20 Years of Fibromyalgia, Jaw Pain and Headaches**
Diagnosis: Fibromyalgia, jaw pain, and headaches
Symptoms: Jaw pain, daily headaches, chronic pain, fatigue and stiffness, low energy, body pain, and jaw clicking.
Previous Failed Treatments: Dentist and medical doctors
Length of Injury: 20 years
Pain Level on a Scale of 0 to 10:
Treatment: Treatment included releasing fibrotic tissue, addressing fascia restrictions, decreasing inflammation, improving ergonomics, implementing an anti-inflammatory diet, and addressing vitamin, mineral, and hormonal

imbalances.
Outcome: Symptoms resolved.

Feel free to scan the QR code below to watch more live treatment cases.

A Biopsychosocial Approach to Beating Migraines

Migraines are not simple headaches nor isolated neurological events. They are a complex, chronic pain disorder shaped by biological vulnerability, nervous system sensitization, mechanical stress, and behavioral patterns that accumulate over time. Conventional migraine treatment has focused primarily on pharmacologic symptom suppression, often without addressing the underlying contributors that lower the migraine threshold and promote chronicity. As a result, many individuals experience temporary relief without meaningful long-term improvement.

The seven natural secrets presented in this book are grounded in a **biopsychosocial model of health**, which recognizes that migraines arise through the interaction of biological dysfunction, psychological stress and nervous system dysregulation, and daily behavioral and mechanical influences. A growing body of research supports this integrative framework, demonstrating that migraines are influenced by neuroinflammation, nutrient status, hormonal balance, posture, connective tissue health, stress physiology, and habitual behaviors (Goadsby et al., 2017). Addressing these contributors together is essential for sustained migraine improvement.

The Biopsychosocial Model Explained

The biopsychosocial model was introduced by George Engel to address the limitations of the traditional biomedical model, which views disease as a purely biological malfunction (Engel, 1977). Rather than isolating pathology to a single organ or mechanism, the biopsychosocial model recognizes that health and illness emerge from the dynamic interaction of multiple systems. Applied to migraines, this model highlights the role of:

1. **Biological factors**, including neuroinflammation, cortical hyperexcitability, mitochondrial dysfunction, micronutrient deficiencies, hormonal fluctuations, vascular instability, and connective tissue restriction
2. **Psychological factors**, such as stress perception, trauma exposure, anxiety, depression, and autonomic nervous system imbalance
3. **Behavioral and social factors**, including posture, movement patterns, sleep regularity, dietary habits, screen exposure, and repetitive daily behaviors

The Biopsychosocial Model for Beating Migraines

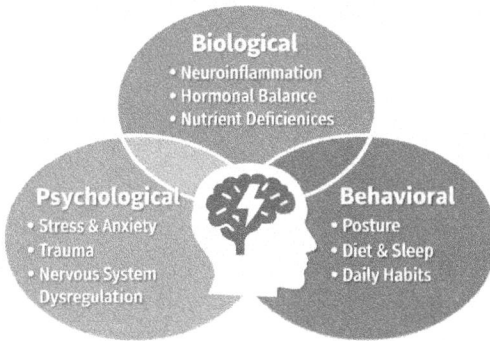

Biological
- Neuroinflammation
- Hormonal Balance
- Nutrient Deficienices

Psychological
- Stress & Anxiety
- Trauma
- Nervous System Dysregulation

Behavioral
- Posture
- Diet & Sleep
- Daily Habits

7 Natural Secrets to Beating Migraines

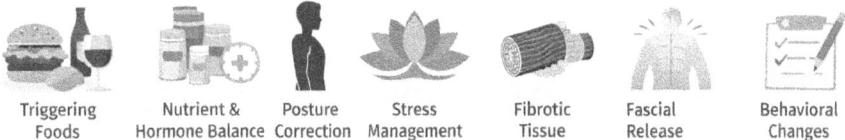

| Triggering Foods | Nutrient & Hormone Balance | Posture Correction | Stress Management | Fibrotic Tissue | Fascial Release | Behavioral Changes |

Migraines exemplify the need for this model, as treating pain alone fails to address the upstream drivers that sensitize the trigeminovascular system and perpetuate recurrent attacks.

1. Migraine-Triggering Foods and Neuroinflammation

Dietary triggers are among the most consistently reported contributors to migraine onset. Certain foods increase neuroinflammation, alter vascular tone, or stimulate excitatory neurotransmitters such as glutamate. Common migraine-triggering foods include aged cheeses, processed meats, alcohol, artificial sweeteners, monosodium glutamate, histamine-rich foods, and highly refined carbohydrates.

Clinical trials demonstrate that individualized elimination of dietary triggers significantly reduces migraine frequency and severity. In a randomized, double-blind crossover study, removing IgG-mediated food triggers resulted in a meaningful reduction in migraine days and symptom burden (Alpay et al., 2010). In addition, whole-food, anti-inflammatory dietary patterns reduce inflammatory mediators and stabilize neuronal excitability, supporting migraine prevention (Gazerani, 2020).

2. Imbalance of Vitamins, Minerals, and Hormones

Micronutrient deficiencies play a central role in migraine pathophysiology. Magnesium deficiency is one of the most well-established contributors, impairing neuronal membrane stability and increasing susceptibility to cortical spreading depression. Multiple clinical studies demonstrate that magnesium supplementation reduces migraine frequency and intensity (Sun-Edelstein & Mauskop, 2009).

Riboflavin (vitamin B2) and coenzyme Q10 support mitochondrial energy production, which is often impaired in individuals with migraines. A randomized controlled trial showed that high-dose riboflavin significantly reduced migraine attack frequency compared to placebo (Schoenen et al., 1998). Vitamin D deficiency has also been associated with increased migraine prevalence, likely through its role in immune regulation and inflammation (Buettner et al., 2015). Hormonal fluctuations, particularly estrogen variability, further influence migraine patterns, explaining the higher prevalence of migraines in women and their association with menstrual cycles, pregnancy, and perimenopause (MacGregor, 2014).

3. Posture and Mechanical Stress on the Nervous System

Postural dysfunction imposes chronic mechanical stress on the cervical spine, cranial nerves, and surrounding soft tissues. Forward head posture and prolonged screen use increase tension in the suboccipital muscles, alter cervical joint mechanics, and compress neurovascular structures involved in migraine pain. Biomechanical studies demonstrate that sustained postural strain alters proprioceptive input to the brain and increases nociceptive signaling. Clinical trials show that cervical rehabilitation and postural correction significantly reduce migraine frequency, intensity, and disability (Fernández-de-Las-Peñas et al., 2006).

4. Stress Management and Autonomic Nervous System Regulation

Stress is one of the most commonly reported migraine triggers and operates through dysregulation of the autonomic nervous system and activation of the hypothalamic-pituitary-adrenal axis. Chronic stress elevates cortisol and catecholamines, alters cerebral blood flow, and sensitizes trigeminal pain pathways. Longitudinal studies demonstrate that individuals with higher perceived stress experience more frequent migraines independent of other factors (Sauro & Becker, 2009). Behavioral interventions that reduce autonomic overactivation, such as biofeedback and mindfulness-based stress reduction, have been shown to significantly reduce migraine frequency and disability (Nestoriuc et al., 2008).

5. Fibrotic Tissue and Chronic Soft Tissue Dysfunction

Chronic inflammation, injury, or repetitive strain leads to the development of fibrotic tissue within muscles and connective structures of the neck, shoulders, and jaw. Fibrotic tissue restricts normal tissue glide, compresses nerves and blood vessels, and perpetuates nociceptive signaling associated with migraines. Research on myofascial pain syndromes demonstrates that treating fibrotic tissue reduces referred pain patterns and improves headache outcomes (Gerwin, 2005). Addressing soft tissue dysfunction reduces peripheral drivers of central sensitization.

6. Fascial Restriction and Force Transmission

Fascia is a continuous connective tissue network that transmits mechanical tension throughout the body. Restrictions in fascial planes of the cervical spine and cranial region alter force distribution and increase strain on migraine-sensitive structures. Emerging evidence confirms that fascial stiffness disrupts neuromuscular coordination and pain modulation. Restoring fascial mobility reduces abnormal tension and improves sensory processing (Stecco et al., 2014).

7. Behavioral Modification and Migraine Threshold

Behavioral patterns ultimately determine whether biological vulnerabilities translate into clinical migraines. Irregular sleep, skipped meals, dehydration, excessive screen exposure, and inconsistent routines destabilize the nervous system and lower the migraine threshold. Prospective studies show that consistent sleep timing, hydration, and daily routines significantly reduce migraine frequency (Penzien et al., 2015). Behavioral migraine management programs demonstrate outcomes comparable to pharmacologic therapy without medication-related side effects.

Conclusion: A Model Built on Science, Not Opinion

The approach outlined in this book is grounded in decades of research across neurology, nutrition science, biomechanics, psychology, and pain physiology. Migraines persist not because they are untreatable, but because they are often addressed too narrowly. The biopsychosocial model provides the framework necessary to understand why migraines become chronic and why isolated interventions frequently fail. Neuroinflammation, nutrient imbalance, hormonal fluctuation, mechanical strain, fascial restriction, stress physiology, and daily behavioral patterns interact continuously to shape migraine threshold and severity. Each of the seven natural secrets targets one of these contributors. Addressed together, they reduce nervous system reactivity and support lasting relief.

Understanding Migraines

Migraines are a complex neurological disorder characterized by recurring episodes of moderate to severe headaches, often accompanied by sensory disturbances. They affect approximately 12% of the global population, with a higher prevalence among women due to hormonal influences (Lipton et al., 2020). Unlike typical headaches, migraines are often debilitating and can interfere with daily functioning. Current research suggests a multifaceted interplay between genetic, environmental, and neurovascular factors in migraine pathophysiology (Goadsby et al., 2017).

Symptoms and Types of Migraines

Migraines present with a wide range of symptoms that can vary between individuals. The hallmark symptom is a unilateral, throbbing headache that intensifies with physical activity and is frequently accompanied by nausea, vomiting, photophobia (sensitivity to light), and phonophobia (sensitivity to sound) (Dodick, 2018). Migraines are typically classified into two main types: migraines with aura and migraines without aura.

Migraines with aura, affecting about one-third of migraine sufferers, involve transient neurological disturbances preceding the headache phase. These disturbances can include visual phenomena such as scintillating scotomas (flashing lights or zigzag patterns), sensory changes like tingling or numbness, and language difficulties (Haanes & Edvinsson, 2019). On the other hand, migraines without aura, which account for the majority of cases, occur without these warning signs and progress directly to the headache phase (Goadsby et al., 2017).

Chronic migraines, defined as headaches occurring on 15 or more days per month for at least three months, represent a more severe form of the disorder (Lipton et al., 2020). These migraines often result from medication overuse, genetic predisposition, and comorbid conditions such as anxiety and depression (Buse et al., 2019).

Biophysiology of Migraines

The underlying biophysiology of migraines involves complex neurovascular and neuroinflammatory mechanisms. One of the primary theories, the "neurovascular hypothesis," suggests that migraines result from abnormal interactions between the brainstem, trigeminal nerve, and intracranial blood vessels (Goadsby et al., 2017). During a migraine attack, the trigeminovascular system becomes activated, leading to the release of pro-inflammatory neuropeptides such as calcitonin gene-related peptide (CGRP), substance P, and neurokinin A, which contribute to vasodilation and inflammation of meningeal blood vessels (Ashina et al., 2021).

Functional neuroimaging studies have also identified the role of cortical spreading depression (CSD) in the pathophysiology of migraines with aura. CSD is a wave of neuronal depolarization followed by suppression of cortical activity, which can trigger the aura phase and subsequent activation of pain pathways (Charles & Baca, 2013). Additionally, dysfunction in serotonin (5-HT) signaling has been implicated in migraine pathogenesis (Dussor, 2022).

Further research suggests that migraines may also involve dysfunctions in the hypothalamus, which regulates circadian rhythms and homeostasis (Schulte & May, 2019). This could explain the common migraine triggers related to sleep disturbances, stress, and hormonal fluctuations. Understanding these biophysiological processes is essential for developing targeted treatments that address both the acute and preventive management of migraines.

Migraines are a complex neurological disorder involving multiple physiological mechanisms. Research indicates that migraines result from an interplay of neurological, vascular, inflammatory, and genetic factors. This disorder affects millions worldwide, with significant implications for daily functioning and quality of life (Goadsby et al., 2017). Advances in neuroscience have provided deeper insights into the biological mechanisms that drive migraines, including the role of the trigeminovascular system, neurotransmitters, cortical spreading depression, inflammation, and genetic predisposition.

The Trigeminovascular System and Neurovascular Activation

One of the key components in migraine pathophysiology is the trigeminovascular system, which is responsible for pain transmission from the meninges to the brain. Activation of this system leads to the release of neuropeptides such as calcitonin gene-related peptide (CGRP), substance P, and neurokinin A, which promote vasodilation and inflammation in the meninges (Ashina et al., 2021).

Cortical Spreading Depression and Aura

For individuals who experience migraines with aura, cortical spreading depression plays a critical role. This phenomenon involves a slow wave of neuronal depolarization across the cerebral cortex, followed by a period of suppressed brain activity. This process is believed to cause the visual disturbances and sensory symptoms that precede migraine pain (Charles & Baca, 2013). Cortical spreading depression may also activate pain pathways, further contributing to migraine symptoms. Additionally, research suggests that this process may weaken the blood-brain barrier, increasing sensitivity to potential migraine triggers (Pietrobon & Moskowitz, 2019).

Neurotransmitters and Their Role in Migraine

Serotonin has long been implicated in migraine pathophysiology. Studies indicate that serotonin levels fluctuate during different phases of a migraine, with a notable drop contributing to vasodilation and pain sensitivity (Dussor, 2022). Dopamine dysregulation has also been linked to migraines, as many individuals report premonitory symptoms such as yawning, mood changes, and drowsiness before an attack, all of which are associated with dopamine fluctuations (Magon & May, 2017).

Brain Structure and Functional Changes

Neuroimaging studies have revealed significant structural and functional changes in the brains of individuals with chronic migraines. The hypothalamus, which regulates sleep, appetite, and circadian rhythms, appears to play a role in the onset of migraines, as hypothalamic activation has been observed before attacks occur (Schulte & May, 2019). Increased connectivity in pain-processing areas, such as the thalamus and periaqueductal gray, suggests that individuals with migraines have heightened sensitivity to pain stimuli (May, 2019). Functional imaging also indicates increased cortical excitability in migraineurs, making their brains more responsive to external stimuli such as bright lights and strong odors (Sprenger & Borsook, 2012).

Inflammation and the Immune System

Emerging evidence suggests that neuroinflammation contributes to migraine pathophysiology. Studies have identified elevated levels of pro-inflammatory cytokines, including tumor necrosis factor-alpha (TNF-α) and interleukin-6 (IL-6), in individuals with migraines (Vecchia & Pietrobon, 2019). Inflammation may also contribute to blood-brain barrier dysfunction, allowing immune cells to enter the brain and sustain chronic migraine conditions (Pietrobon & Moskowitz, 2019). Anti-inflammatory treatments and dietary interventions aimed at reducing systemic inflammation have shown promise in migraine management.

Genetic and Epigenetic Contributions

Genetic studies have shown that migraines have a strong hereditary component, with approximately 50% heritability. Genome-wide association studies have identified multiple genes linked to migraine susceptibility, particularly those involved in ion channel function and neurotransmitter regulation (Ferrari et al., 2015). Additionally, environmental factors such as stress, diet, and inflammation may modify gene expression, increasing migraine susceptibility in certain individuals (Gormley et al., 2016).

Conclusion

Migraines involve complex neurological and vascular processes, with significant contributions from neurotransmitters, inflammation, and genetics. The activation of the trigeminovascular system, cortical spreading depression, and changes in serotonin levels all play a role in the development of migraine attacks. However, migraines are not just a neurological condition—they are also influenced by lifestyle factors, diet, posture, stress levels, and environmental toxins. By addressing these contributing factors through a holistic, multi-faceted approach, it is possible to break the cycle of chronic migraines and support the body's natural ability to heal. The seven elements I present in this book address the root causes of migraines holistically, focusing on both prevention and long-term relief.

Navigating The Healing Journey: How Your Body Recovers Naturally

Migraine is a prevalent neurological disorder affecting a significant portion of the global population. Recent estimates suggest that approximately 14–15% of individuals worldwide experience migraines, accounting for 4.9% of global population ill health (Steiner & Stovner, 2023). In the United States, the prevalence has remained relatively stable over the past three decades, ranging from 11.7% to 14.7% overall, with higher rates observed in women (17.1% to 19.2%) compared to men (5.6% to 7.2%) (Burch et al., 2022). Globally, migraine affects more than one billion individuals each year, making it one of the most common neurologic disorders, particularly among young adults and females

Normal Healing Cycle

Inflammation

Increased Temperature
Loss of Function
Redness
Swelling
Pain

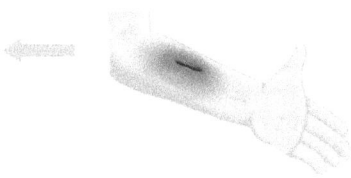

Proliferation

Fibrosis (Scar Tissue)
Fascia Restriction
Muscle Spasm
Trigger Points

Maturation

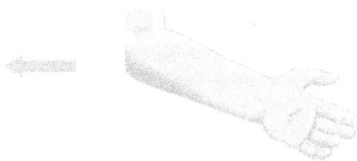

ASTR

(Ashina et al., 2021). The burden of migraine is substantial, contributing to significant disability and impacting individuals' quality of life.

Understanding the normal body healing process is essential for effectively treating migraines, as migraines are often linked to systemic imbalances, inflammation, and impaired recovery mechanisms. The body's natural healing cycle involves recognition, response, repair, and restoration. When an injury or imbalance occurs, the body initiates an inflammatory response to address the issue, followed by cellular repair and tissue regeneration. However, chronic migraines may result from dysregulated healing processes, where persistent inflammation, nervous system hypersensitivity, and vascular dysfunction interfere with the body's ability to restore balance. These disruptions prevent normal recovery, leading to recurring migraine attacks and prolonged discomfort.

Research suggests that individuals with migraines often exhibit impaired mitochondrial function, oxidative stress, and neurovascular dysregulation, which can hinder normal healing mechanisms. These disruptions can contribute to prolonged pain cycles and increased migraine frequency. Understanding how the body heals and identifying factors that interfere with this process, such as nutrient deficiencies, chronic stress, and myofascial restrictions, are essential for effective treatment. By implementing targeted strategies, recovery can be enhanced, inflammation reduced, and neurological balance restored. Addressing these underlying dysfunctions through dietary modifications, stress management, and manual therapies can help optimize the body's healing cycle and improve migraine outcomes.

The normal healing cycle consists of three stages, which can be illustrated using an external paper cut to visualize what happens internally in the body. See the image above for more details. The first stage is inflammation, characterized by swelling, redness, pain, and increased blood flow to the affected area. The second stage involves the formation of fibrosis, also known as scar tissue, which fills the wound to prevent it from remaining open and susceptible to infection. During this stage, the injured site may also experience fascial restrictions and muscle spasms. This highlights the essential role of scar tissue in our protection and survival.

The third stage of the healing cycle involves the breakdown of fibrotic tissue. Ideally, in a perfect world with perfect bodies, the body would autonomously break down this fibrotic tissue over a period of days, weeks, or months, depending on the severity of the injury. However, we do not live in a perfect world. As we age, our body's ability to break down scar tissue decreases significantly.

This healing process also occurs internally when our bodies experience injuries from accidents, surgeries, trauma, poor posture, or stress. Below, the normal muscle healing process after injury is described in more depth, outlining a complex sequence that can be divided into several overlapping phases. The duration of each phase can vary depending on the severity of the injury and the individual's overall health. In chronic conditions, the injured area may not progress through all three stages, instead getting stuck between the inflammation and proliferation stages. Here is a breakdown of the normal muscle healing cycle:

Destruction Stage (Injury Initiation)

This initial phase begins immediately after injury and is characterized by the disruption of muscle fibers and blood vessels, leading to the formation of a hematoma (a localized collection of blood outside of blood vessels). The hematoma serves to contain the damage and forms a scaffold for incoming inflammatory cells.

1. Inflammatory Stage
This phase starts within hours after the injury and can last for several days. It involves the following key processes:

- **Inflammation**: In response to injury, inflammatory cells such as neutrophils and macrophages infiltrate the site. They remove debris, damaged cells, and pathogens. This phase is associated with the classic signs of inflammation: redness, heat, swelling, and pain.
- **Release of Cytokines**: Inflammatory cells release cytokines and growth factors that are crucial for healing and recruiting more reparative cells to the injury site.

2. Proliferation Stage

During this phase, the focus shifts from clearing out the debris to rebuilding muscle tissue, and typically lasts from several days to a couple of weeks:

- **Myogenesis**: This is the formation of new muscle fibers through the activation, differentiation, and fusion of myoblasts (muscle progenitor cells).
- **Fibroblast Proliferation**: Fibroblasts produce collagen and other extracellular matrix components that form the scar tissue, providing structural integrity to the healing muscle. During this stage, fibrosis (scar tissue) closes the injured site and adheres the fascial layers together, causing fascial restrictions. I will discuss fascial restrictions in depth in the chapter on fascial restriction.
- **Angiogenesis**: New blood vessels form to provide necessary nutrients and oxygen to the regenerating tissue.

3. Maturation Stage: The Remodeling Phase

This final phase can last from several weeks to months and is focused on strengthening and refining the newly formed tissue:

- **Maturation of Muscle Fibers**: Newly formed muscle fibers mature and increase in size and strength.
- **Collagen Remodeling**: The initially disorganized collagen fibers become more organized and aligned along the lines of stress, which improves the tensile strength of the muscle.
- **Functional Recovery**: Gradually, the muscle regains its strength and functionality, although the healed muscle may never completely return to its pre-injury state.

Factors Influencing Muscle Healing

Several factors can affect the efficiency and outcome of muscle healing, including:

- **Age**: Younger individuals tend to heal faster than older adults.
- **Malnutrition**
- **Vitamins, Minerals, and Hormonal Imbalances**
- **Blood Supply**: Muscles with good blood supply generally heal better than those with less vascularization.

- **Re-injury**: Avoiding re-injury during the healing process is crucial for successful recovery.
- **Poor Posture and Body Mechanics**

Chronic Condition Vicious Cycle

According to the U.S. National Center for Health Statistics, a chronic condition is typically defined as one that persists for three months or more. In a chronic condition, the injured body part becomes trapped in a vicious cycle, continuously oscillating between the inflammation and proliferation stages. This cycle leads to excessive inflammation and fibrosis, which in turn cause muscle spasms and severe fascial restrictions. Deficiencies in vitamins and minerals can cause the body to remain stuck in the inflammation-proliferation cycle, preventing progression to the maturation stage. Additionally, excessive fibrosis and severe fascial restrictions can further complicate the issue, making it harder to break the cycle of chronic conditions.

When essential nutrients are lacking, the body's ability to regulate inflammation, repair tissues, and restore normal function is compromised. Deficiencies in key vitamins and minerals disrupt cellular energy production, weaken the immune system, and impair the body's ability to detoxify, further fueling chronic inflammation.

Chronic stress further exacerbates this cycle by increasing cortisol levels, which can dysregulate the immune system, disrupt hormone balance, and intensify inflammation. Elevated stress hormones place the nervous system in a constant state of overactivity, making the body more susceptible to pain and reducing its ability to recover from migraine episodes. Additionally, poor posture and musculoskeletal imbalances contribute to fascial restrictions and tension, further stimulating pain pathways and delaying the body's transition to the maturation stage of healing.

The maturation stage is the final phase of tissue repair, where collagen is properly remodeled, inflammation subsides, and the body fully recovers. However, without sufficient vitamins, minerals, and targeted interventions, the body remains stuck in a state of chronic dysfunction, unable to complete the

Chronic Conditions

Inflammation

Increased Temperature
Loss of Function
Redness
Swelling
Pain

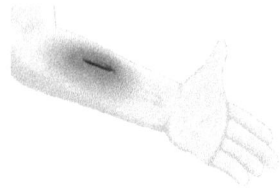

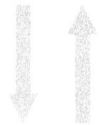

Proliferation

Fibrosis (Scar Tissue)
Fascia Restriction
Muscle Spasm
Trigger Points

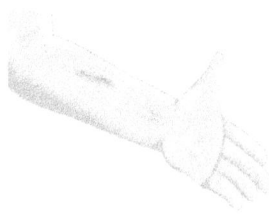

ASTR

healing cycle. Instead of progressing to full recovery, the body continuously cycles through inflammation and proliferation, leading to persistent pain, tissue dysfunction, and ongoing migraine episodes.

In order to break this vicious cycle and effectively treat migraines, it is essential to address the seven elements presented in this book, which are designed to restore balance, reduce inflammation, and promote long-term healing. By optimizing nutrition, correcting postural imbalances, managing stress, and supporting the body's natural healing mechanisms, individuals can transition from chronic pain and inflammation to full recovery and neurological stability. Properly nourishing the body with the right balance of vitamins and minerals is a crucial step in allowing it to move beyond the inflammatory phase and complete the healing process.

Migraine-Triggering Foods

Migraine-Triggering Foods: Understanding the Dietary Connection

Migraines are a complex neurological condition with multiple contributing factors, and diet plays a crucial role in both triggering and preventing attacks. Research has consistently shown that certain foods and beverages can increase migraine frequency and severity in susceptible individuals (Sun-Edelstein & Mauskop, 2009). While triggers vary from person to person, several common dietary culprits have been identified. Through my own experience with migraines, I discovered that coffee, pasteurized dairy products (but not raw dairy), and alcohol were significant triggers. Over the years, I have worked with many patients who also identified multiple food triggers that contributed to their migraines. Below, I explore the most common migraine-inducing foods based on both scientific research and clinical experience.

Processed Meats and Nitrates

Processed meats such as bacon, ham, hot dogs, sausage, and deli meats contain nitrates and nitrites, preservatives used to enhance color and prolong shelf life. These compounds have been shown to cause vasodilation, which can trigger migraines in sensitive individuals (Ramadan, 2018). A study by Lippi et al. (2016) found a significant association between dietary nitrates and increased migraine occurrence, suggesting that reducing consumption of these foods may help lower migraine risk.

Aged Cheeses and Tyramine

Aged cheeses like cheddar, blue cheese, gouda, parmesan, and Swiss contain tyramine, a naturally occurring compound formed as proteins break down over time. Tyramine can influence blood pressure and cerebral blood flow, both of which have been implicated in migraine pathophysiology (de Roos et al., 2017). Research indicates that individuals with reduced ability to metabolize tyramine may be more prone to migraine attacks following consumption of aged cheeses (Finocchi & Sivori, 2012).

Alcohol

Alcohol, particularly red wine, beer, and champagne, has been a personal migraine trigger for me, and I have seen the same pattern in many of my patients. The exact mechanism remains unclear, but possible explanations include histamine and tannin content, dehydration, and alcohol-induced fluctuations in serotonin levels (Martin et al., 2016). Red wine, in particular, contains high levels of histamines and sulfites, both of which have been linked to migraine onset (Janse et al., 2020). Studies suggest that even small amounts of alcohol can provoke migraines in sensitive individuals, making avoidance a key strategy for those prone to attacks.

Artificial Sweeteners

Aspartame, commonly found in diet sodas, sugar-free gums, and low-calorie snacks, has been implicated in migraine attacks due to its effects on neurotransmitters and oxidative stress (Bigal & Krymchantowski, 2006). Research by Humphrey et al. (2008) found that aspartame consumption was associated with increased headache frequency, particularly in individuals with a history of migraines. Sucralose, another artificial sweetener, has also been reported to provoke headaches in some individuals.

Caffeine

For years, I relied on coffee, unaware that it was one of my biggest migraine triggers. Caffeine has a paradoxical effect on migraines—it can help relieve migraines in some cases but also trigger them when consumed excessively or withdrawn suddenly (Rogers et al., 2016). While moderate caffeine intake can constrict blood vessels and provide temporary relief, habitual overconsumption can lead to caffeine dependency and rebound headaches when intake is reduced. The American Migraine Foundation recommends limiting caffeine intake to no more than 200 mg per day to avoid dependency-related migraines (Lipton et al., 2017).

Chocolate

Chocolate is one of the most commonly reported migraine triggers, affecting nearly 22% of migraine sufferers (Nicolodi & Sicuteri, 1999). It contains tyramine, histamine, caffeine, and phenylethylamine, all of which may contribute to migraines in sensitive individuals. Studies suggest that chocolate-induced migraines may be partially attributed to serotonin fluctuations and inflammatory responses in the brain (Hoffmann & Recober, 2013).

MSG and Additives

Monosodium glutamate (MSG), a common food additive found in processed snacks, fast food, instant noodles, and canned soups, has been linked to migraines and headaches (Shimomura et al., 2019). Research suggests that MSG can trigger migraines by overactivating glutamate receptors in the brain, leading to neuroexcitotoxicity and inflammation (Ribiero et al., 2018). Avoiding foods labeled with "flavor enhancer," "hydrolyzed protein," or "yeast extract" may help reduce MSG-related migraines.

High-Sugar and High-Glycemic Foods

Refined carbohydrates and high-sugar foods, including pastries, white bread, and sugary drinks, can cause rapid spikes and crashes in blood sugar levels, which may trigger migraines (Hungerbühler et al., 2016). A study by Martins et al. (2021) found that individuals consuming high-glycemic diets had a greater frequency of migraines, highlighting the importance of blood sugar regulation in migraine prevention.

Pasteurized Dairy

Through my personal experience and working with patients, I have found that pasteurized dairy products, including milk, yogurt, and cheese, can be a significant migraine trigger. Unlike raw dairy, which retains its natural enzymes, pasteurized dairy may contribute to migraines due to casein protein intolerance, lactose sensitivity, or inflammation caused by dairy processing (Aragón et al., 2020). Many of my patients have reported improvements in their migraine symptoms after eliminating pasteurized dairy from their diet.

Nuts and Seeds

Certain nuts and seeds, including walnuts, peanuts, almonds, and sunflower seeds, are high in arginine, an amino acid that can influence nitric oxide production and cause blood vessel dilation, potentially leading to migraines (Sarchielli et al., 2012). While nuts provide essential nutrients, individuals sensitive to arginine may benefit from reducing their intake.

Dehydration as a Migraine Trigger

Dehydration is a well-documented trigger for migraines, as even mild fluid deficits can lead to physiological changes that contribute to headache onset. Water plays a crucial role in maintaining vascular stability, electrolyte balance, and optimal brain function. When dehydration occurs, the body experiences a reduction in blood volume, leading to cerebral vasodilation and increased osmolarity, both of which have been linked to migraine pathophysiology (Yoshimoto et al., 2020). A study by Lippi et al. (2020) found that dehydration-related migraines are often associated with electrolyte imbalances, particularly sodium and potassium disturbances, which affect neuronal excitability and pain perception.

Neurological studies suggest that dehydration can contribute to central sensitization, a condition where the nervous system becomes more responsive to stimuli, increasing migraine susceptibility (Dussor, 2022). Dehydration also affects serotonin and histamine levels, both of which play roles in migraine initiation. In a study by Spigt et al. (2012), migraine sufferers who increased their daily water intake experienced a significant reduction in headache intensity and frequency, reinforcing the importance of hydration in migraine prevention. Additionally, a study by Ramadan et al. (2015) found that individuals who maintained consistent hydration had a lower risk of developing migraines, as dehydration can exacerbate inflammatory pathways and trigger neurovascular disturbances.

The relationship between dehydration and migraines is particularly significant in individuals exposed to high temperatures, excessive caffeine consumption, or prolonged physical activity, all of which increase the risk of fluid loss. Many migraine sufferers also fail to recognize the early signs of dehydration, such as dizziness, dry mouth, and fatigue, which can precede the onset of a migraine attack (Lippi et al., 2020). Given the strong link between hydration and migraine prevention, maintaining adequate fluid intake is a simple yet effective strategy to help reduce the frequency and severity of migraines.

For me, pasteurized dairy products, coffee, processed food, and alcohol trigger migraines. Unfortunately, I used to drink coffee and consume pasteurized dairy products daily, unaware of their potential impact on my health. It is very common for migraine sufferers to unknowingly consume their trigger foods on a regular basis, making it difficult to identify the exact cause of their headaches. Many individuals continue eating the same foods, unaware that they may be contributing to chronic inflammation, neurotransmitter imbalances, and vascular instability, all of which can play a role in migraine onset.

While food triggers vary from person to person, research suggests that migraines are rarely caused by a single dietary factor. Instead, most migraine sufferers have multiple triggers, often five to seven, including dietary, environmental, and lifestyle influences. For example, factors such as stress, dehydration, hormonal fluctuations, and poor sleep can amplify the effects of food-based triggers. Through my own journey with migraines and years of clinical experience, I have seen the profound impact that dietary changes can have on reducing migraine frequency and severity. Identifying personal triggers requires patience and a strategic approach, such as keeping a food journal and following an elimination diet. By systematically removing and reintroducing potential trigger foods, individuals can better understand how their body reacts to specific ingredients. This process helps them create a sustainable, migraine-friendly eating plan that promotes long-term relief and overall health.

Medication-overuse headache

This section does not focus on foods that may trigger migraines but instead provides valuable information about medications that could contribute to headaches. Research has shown that certain medications, particularly analgesics and vasodilators, can trigger or exacerbate headaches. A study by Scher et al. (2017) found that frequent use of over-the-counter pain relievers, such as ibuprofen and acetaminophen, increases the risk of medication-overuse headaches (MOH). This condition occurs when excessive reliance on painkillers leads to rebound headaches, making migraines more frequent and difficult to manage.

Similarly, nitrates and other vasodilators used to treat cardiovascular conditions have been associated with headache induction due to their ability to dilate blood vessels, as reported by Silvestrini et al. (2019). Furthermore, hormonal medications, including oral contraceptives, have been linked to an increased risk of migraines, particularly in individuals with a history of migraine with aura (MacGregor, 2020). Understanding the impact of medications on headache development is crucial for effective migraine management.

Medication-Overuse Headache and Medication-Induced Migraine

Medication-overuse headache (MOH) is a paradoxical condition characterized by the increased frequency and severity of headaches due to the overuse of headache-relief medications (Goadsby et al., 2002). This cyclical pattern arises as the body becomes dependent on the medication, leading to rebound headaches when the medication is not taken, thus necessitating more medication for relief, ultimately exacerbating the headache problem (Diener et al., 2018).

Medication-Overuse Headache (MOH)

MOH diagnosis relies on a detailed headache history, medication usage patterns, and often, symptom improvement after cessation of the offending medication (Headache Classification Committee of the International Headache Society, 2018). Differentiating MOH from other headache disorders is crucial for effective management.

Offending Medications and Usage Frequency: The risk of MOH is associated with both the type of medication and the frequency of use. Specific criteria for overuse include:

- **Triptans (e.g., sumatriptan, rizatriptan):** Use on 10 or more days per month (Ferrari et al., 2017).
- **Opioids (e.g., codeine, hydrocodone):** Use on 10 or more days per month (Bigal et al., 2008).
- **Ergotamines (e.g., ergotamine, dihydroergotamine):** Use on 10 or more days per month (Goadsby et al., 2002).
- **Combination Analgesics (e.g., medications containing a combination of a pain reliever, caffeine, and/or a barbiturate):** Use on 10 or more days per month (Lipton et al., 2005).

- **Simple Analgesics (e.g., acetaminophen, aspirin, ibuprofen, naproxen):** Use on 15 or more days per month (Schulman et al., 2019).

Symptoms of MOH: MOH often presents as a chronic daily or near-daily headache. The pain characteristics may mirror the original headache type or differ. Additional symptoms can include increased headache frequency and severity, diminished medication effectiveness, nausea, restlessness, and difficulty concentrating (Tfelt-Hansen et al., 2010).

Medications that Can Trigger or Worsen Migraines (Beyond MOH)

Beyond MOH, certain medications can trigger or exacerbate migraines even with infrequent use.

- **Nitroglycerin:** This medication, used for angina, is a known migraine trigger in susceptible individuals due to its vasodilatory effects (Limmroth et al., 2002).
- **Hormonal Medications (e.g., Oral Contraceptives, Hormone Replacement Therapy):** Hormonal fluctuations, particularly estrogen level changes, can significantly influence migraine patterns (MacGregor et al., 2010). Hormonal birth control can sometimes improve migraines, but it can also worsen them or initiate new-onset migraines.

Other Potential Triggers: While not always definitively established, other medications may be potential migraine triggers in some individuals. These include certain blood pressure medications, some antidepressants, and some medications for heart conditions.

How to Identify Your Personal Migraine Triggers

Since migraines are highly individualized, it is essential to systematically test and identify which foods may be triggering your symptoms. Many people have more than three food-related migraine triggers, making it important to approach the process with patience and a structured plan. Below are some practical steps to help pinpoint and eliminate foods that could be contributing to your migraines.

1. Keep a Detailed Food and Migraine Journal

Tracking what you eat and how you feel afterward is one of the most effective ways to identify potential food triggers. Use a notebook or a mobile app to record:

- Everything you eat and drink, including portion sizes and ingredients.
- The time of day you eat each meal or snack.
- Any migraine symptoms that occur, including their intensity and duration.
- Other factors such as stress levels, hydration, sleep quality, and physical activity.

Over time, patterns may emerge, helping you link certain foods to migraine episodes.

2. ASTR Diet: Try an Elimination Diet

The **ASTR Diet** helps identify and eliminate migraine-triggering foods while promoting long-term healing through an anti-inflammatory, toxin-free, and restorative approach. An elimination diet is an effective method for pinpointing food-related migraine triggers and reducing the frequency and intensity of attacks.

To follow the ASTR elimination diet effectively:

- **Remove all potential migraine triggers** at once for a set period (typically 3-4 days). This includes processed meats, aged cheeses, alcohol, caffeine, artificial sweeteners, MSG, chocolate, high-glycemic foods, pasteurized dairy, and nuts.
- **Focus on whole, unprocessed foods** that nourish the body and reduce inflammation. Prioritize fresh vegetables, proteins, healthy fats, and nutrient-dense foods to support healing.
- **Reintroduce foods systematically** after the elimination phase. If migraines improve after 3-4 days, begin adding back one eliminated food at a time, waiting at least 1-2 days before introducing another.
- **Monitor symptoms closely.** If a migraine occurs after reintroducing a food, that food may be a trigger and should be avoided or limited in the long term.

Following the ASTR Diet's elimination approach helps individuals understand their unique migraine triggers and take proactive steps to heal naturally while maintaining a balanced, nutrient-rich diet. However, due to the complexity of the ASTR Diet and the many factors involved in its implementation, it is challenging to cover all aspects in just a few pages. The diet is designed not only to reduce migraine triggers but also to support overall health through an anti-inflammatory, sustainable, toxin-free, and restorative approach. To learn more about the ASTR Diet, including how to implement it effectively for migraine relief and long-term wellness, refer to my book *Eat to Heal*, which provides a comprehensive guide to this nutritional strategy.

3. Test Each Food Individually

Instead of removing multiple foods at once, some people prefer to test foods one by one to see if they provoke migraines. To do this:

- Choose a food from the list of common migraine triggers and eat a small amount.
- Monitor symptoms for 24-48 hours, as some food reactions can be delayed.
- If no reaction occurs, gradually increase the portion over a few days to confirm tolerance.
- If a migraine occurs, remove that food and wait a few days before testing another.

4. Be Cautious When Testing Dairy

Pasteurized dairy, in particular, can be tricky to test because reactions can vary depending on the type and source of dairy. If you suspect dairy might be a trigger:

- Start with **small amounts** of dairy, such as a spoonful of yogurt or a slice of cheese.
- Note whether different forms of dairy (milk, cheese, yogurt) cause symptoms.
- If pasteurized dairy triggers migraines, but raw dairy does not, this could indicate sensitivity to processing changes rather than the dairy itself.
- Some people tolerate certain dairy types better (e.g., goat's milk instead of cow's milk).

5. Consider Combining Testing with Other Lifestyle Factors

Sometimes food triggers interact with stress, dehydration, poor sleep, or hormonal fluctuations, making it difficult to pinpoint a single cause. If you're testing foods, try to maintain a consistent routine in other areas of your life to get clearer results.

Conclusion

Most people with food-related migraines have **more than three dietary triggers**, meaning a single elimination may not be enough to provide full relief. By systematically testing and identifying problem foods, you can create a personalized migraine-friendly diet that works best for your body. While this process takes time, it can lead to significant improvements in migraine frequency, severity, and overall well-being. If you suspect food is playing a role in your migraines but struggle to identify specific triggers, working with nutritionist familiar with migraine diets can provide additional guidance.

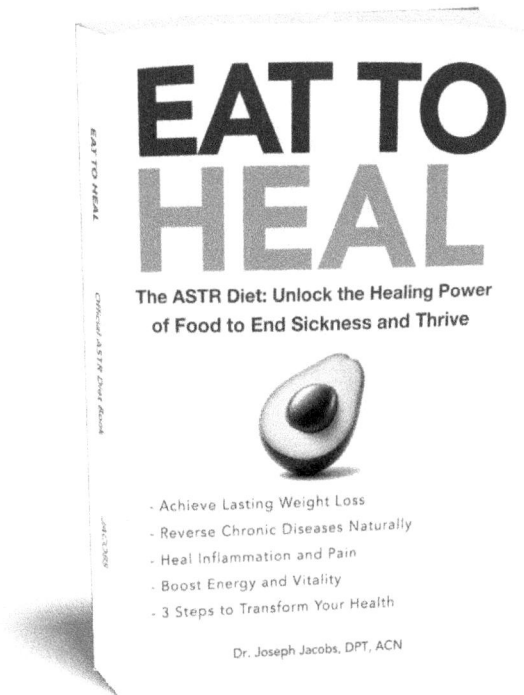

EAT TO HEAL

The ASTR Diet: Unlock the Healing Power of Food to End Sickness and Thrive

- Achieve Lasting Weight Loss
- Reverse Chronic Diseases Naturally
- Heal Inflammation and Pain
- Boost Energy and Vitality
- 3 Steps to Transform Your Health

Dr. Joseph Jacobs, DPT, ACN

Imbalance of Vitamins, Minerals, and Hormones

The Role of Vitamin, Mineral, and Hormonal Deficiencies in Migraines

Migraines are a complex neurological disorder influenced by various factors, including deficiencies in specific vitamins, minerals, and hormones. Research has identified several nutrient deficiencies that may contribute to the onset and severity of migraine attacks. However, because each individual's biochemistry is unique, it is essential to work with a **clinical nutritionist** to conduct **comprehensive lab testing** to identify specific deficiencies and determine the appropriate dosage of supplementation. Treating migraines effectively requires a **customized** approach, as lab values and nutritional needs differ from person to person.

Vitamin D Deficiency

Vitamin D plays a critical role in modulating inflammation and maintaining neuronal health. A deficiency in vitamin D has been associated with an increased risk of migraines. A study by Ghorbani et al. (2019) found that individuals with lower serum levels of vitamin D experienced longer durations of migraine headaches, suggesting that inadequate vitamin D levels contribute to prolonged migraine attacks. Further research indicates that vitamin D influences the immune system and inflammatory pathways, which are often dysregulated in migraine sufferers. Proper supplementation, based on individual lab results, may help reduce migraine frequency and intensity (*Ghorbani et al., 2019*). Optimal dosing requires lab-guided monitoring, as excessive vitamin D may lead to hypercalcemia, kidney strain, and increased cardiovascular risk.

Magnesium Deficiency

Magnesium is essential for numerous physiological processes, including neuromuscular function and neurotransmitter regulation. Low magnesium levels have been linked to increased neuronal excitability, a factor implicated in migraine pathogenesis. Research indicates that magnesium deficiency is common among migraine sufferers, and lower serum magnesium levels are correlated with increased migraine frequency and severity (*Mauskop & Varughese, 2012*). A double-blind study found that magnesium supplementation reduced migraine attacks by up to 41%, further confirming its role in migraine prevention (*Peikert et al., 1996*). However, excessive magnesium intake can cause gastrointestinal distress, making personalized dosing through lab testing essential.

Riboflavin (Vitamin B2) Deficiency

Riboflavin is crucial for mitochondrial energy production, and mitochondrial dysfunction has been proposed as a contributing factor in migraines. A systematic review of randomized controlled trials concluded that riboflavin supplementation significantly reduced the frequency and duration of migraines (*Thompson et al., 2017*). Because riboflavin is water-soluble, excess amounts are excreted in urine, making it a generally safe option. However, optimal dosing should be based on individual laboratory findings to ensure effective levels without unnecessary supplementation.

Cobalamin (Vitamin B12) Deficiency

Vitamin B12, also known as cobalamin, is essential for neurological function and red blood cell formation. Emerging research suggests a potential link between vitamin B12 deficiency and migraine prevalence. A study by Üstün Özek (2022) found that patients with chronic migraines had significantly lower vitamin B12 levels compared to those with less frequent migraine attacks. This negative correlation indicates that vitamin B12 deficiency may contribute to increased migraine frequency and severity.

Similarly, a case-control study by Ghorbani et al. (2019) reported that migraine patients exhibited significantly lower serum vitamin B12 levels and higher methylmalonic acid (MMA) levels, a marker of B12 deficiency, compared to healthy controls. These findings suggest that lower functional activity of vitamin B12 is associated with a higher likelihood of experiencing migraines.

Furthermore, research indicates that vitamin B12 deficiency may be linked to various types of headaches, including tension-type and unclassified headaches. A study by Ayanoğlu et al. (2021) concluded that vitamin B12 levels below 400 pg/mL could be an independent risk factor for these headache disorders in children and adolescents.

Collectively, these studies underscore the importance of assessing vitamin B12 status in individuals suffering from migraines and other headache disorders. Regular monitoring and appropriate supplementation of vitamin B12 may serve as a beneficial component in the holistic management of migraine patients. Excessive intake may cause numbness, burning sensations, and itching, emphasizing the need for personalized dosing.

Vitamin B6 (Pyridoxine) Deficiency

Vitamin B6 plays a crucial role in neurotransmitter synthesis, including serotonin and dopamine, which influence pain regulation and neurological function. Research has indicated that a deficiency in vitamin B6 may contribute to increased migraine susceptibility due to its role in reducing inflammation and modulating homocysteine levels.

A randomized controlled trial by Sadeghi et al. (2015) investigated the effects of pyridoxine supplementation on migraine characteristics. The study found that supplementation significantly reduced the severity and duration of migraine attacks and decreased headache-related disability. These findings suggest that adequate vitamin B6 intake may serve as a beneficial strategy in migraine prevention and management.

Another study using data from the National Health and Nutrition Examination Survey (NHANES) found that individuals with higher dietary intake of vitamin B6 had a reduced risk of experiencing severe headaches or migraines. This suggests that maintaining sufficient levels of pyridoxine through diet or supplementation may be protective against migraines. Excessive intake of vitamin B6 may lead to nerve damage, numbness, and tingling in the hands and feet, highlighting the importance of personalized dosing.

Folate (Vitamin B9) Deficiency

Folate is an essential B vitamin involved in DNA synthesis, red blood cell formation, and homocysteine metabolism. Elevated homocysteine levels have been associated with increased inflammation and vascular dysfunction, both of which are implicated in migraine pathophysiology.

A study by Zhao et al. (2024) observed a significant inverse relationship between dietary folate intake and the prevalence of severe headaches or migraines. Individuals with higher folate consumption had a lower risk of experiencing migraines, emphasizing the potential role of folate in reducing migraine occurrence.

Additionally, research published in the *British Journal of Nutrition* in 2024 found that adults with higher dietary folate intake were less likely to report severe headaches or migraines. These findings highlight the importance of adequate folate intake in supporting vascular health and neurological function, potentially reducing migraine risk. Excessive intake of vitamin B9 may mask vitamin B12 deficiency and contribute to neurological damage, underscoring the importance of personalized dosing.

Coenzyme Q10 (CoQ10) Deficiency

Coenzyme Q10 (CoQ10) is a vital antioxidant involved in mitochondrial energy production. A deficiency in CoQ10 has been observed in individuals with migraines, particularly those with mitochondrial dysfunction. A clinical study found that CoQ10 supplementation led to a significant reduction in migraine frequency and severity within three months (*Hershey et al., 2007*). Since CoQ10 levels naturally decline with age and can be depleted by medications like statins, individualized testing is necessary to determine proper supplementation.

Iron Deficiency

Iron is essential for oxygen transport and energy production. A study by Özdemir et al. (2018) found that low ferritin levels were significantly associated with an increased risk of migraines, particularly in menstruating women. Iron deficiency anemia can lead to hypoxia (low oxygen levels), which may contribute to migraine attacks. However, excess iron can be harmful, leading to oxidative stress and organ damage. Proper lab testing is crucial to assess iron levels before supplementation.

Zinc Deficiency

Zinc is a critical mineral involved in immune function, neurotransmitter activity, and inflammation regulation. Recent studies suggest that low zinc levels may contribute to migraine susceptibility by affecting neuroinflammatory pathways (*Yabanlı & Özer, 2022*). Zinc supplementation has shown promise in migraine prevention, but excess intake can interfere with copper absorption, highlighting the importance of individualized lab assessments.

Estrogen and Progesterone Imbalances

Hormonal fluctuations, particularly in estrogen and progesterone levels, are well-known migraine triggers, especially in women. Estrogen influences vascular function and neurotransmitter activity, which are both implicated in migraine pathophysiology. Research by Martin & Behbehani (2006) found that estrogen withdrawal (as seen in menstrual migraines) can lead to increased migraine frequency and severity. Additionally, low progesterone levels relative to estrogen (estrogen dominance) may further contribute to migraines. Hormone testing can help determine whether dietary modifications, or lifestyle interventions are necessary for balancing hormones and reducing migraine attacks.

Thyroid Hormone Imbalances

Hypothyroidism (low thyroid hormone levels) has been associated with an increased risk of chronic migraines. A study by *Gökmen-Yıldırım et al. (2020)* found that individuals with hypothyroidism had a significantly higher prevalence of migraines compared to those with normal thyroid function. The exact mechanism remains unclear, but thyroid dysfunction may contribute to migraines through metabolic dysregulation and impaired neurotransmitter function. Proper thyroid function testing, including TSH, free T3, free T4, is essential for determining whether thyroid imbalances contribute to migraines.

Cortisol Dysregulation (Adrenal Imbalance)

Cortisol, the primary stress hormone, plays a role in inflammation, pain perception, and energy metabolism. Chronic stress and dysregulated cortisol levels can lead to increased migraine frequency (*Peres et al., 2017*). Low cortisol levels (adrenal fatigue) can impair the body's ability to handle stress, while excessively high cortisol levels contribute to systemic inflammation and vascular dysfunction.

Conclusion

Addressing deficiencies in vitamins, minerals, and hormones through comprehensive lab testing and individualized supplementation is a powerful strategy for managing migraines naturally. While generalized supplementation may help some individuals, a personalized approach based on lab values ensures that the right nutrients are provided at the correct dosages. Working with a clinical nutritionist provider is essential for developing a targeted plan that meets each individual's unique biochemical needs. By identifying and correcting nutrient and hormonal imbalances, individuals can take a proactive approach to reducing migraine frequency, severity, and duration.

Targeted supplementation and dietary modifications can help restore balance in the body, improve neurological function, and reduce inflammation, key factors in migraine prevention. Since deficiencies in vitamins such as vitamin D, riboflavin, and CoQ10, as well as minerals like magnesium and iron, have been linked to migraines, correcting these imbalances may lead to significant symptom improvement. From my clinical experience, migraine patients typically suffer from at least **three to six vitamin and mineral deficiencies**. Additionally, optimizing hormonal health, particularly estrogen and thyroid function, plays a crucial role in stabilizing migraine patterns.

From my personal experience, I struggled with severe deficiencies in B vitamins, vitamin D, magnesium and zinc, which significantly impacted my health and contributed to my migraines. Through comprehensive lab testing, I was able to identify these deficiencies and implement the correct treatment. Evaluating my own lab results allowed me to determine the proper dosage and form of supplementation, which played a crucial role in my recovery. This personalized approach helped me regain balance, eliminate migraines, and enhance my overall well-being.

A well-structured plan that includes lab testing, tailored supplementation, and lifestyle adjustments empowers individuals to regain control over their health and minimize migraine attacks naturally. Long-term migraine management is not just about symptom relief but also about addressing the underlying physiological imbalances that contribute to their occurrence. With proper guidance and a commitment to individualized care, migraine sufferers can experience lasting improvements in their overall well-being and quality of life.

Posture

Poor Neck Posture and Migraines: The Postural Connection

Poor posture, particularly involving the neck, has been implicated in the development and exacerbation of migraines. Forward head posture (FHP), characterized by the anterior positioning of the head relative to the spine, is a common postural deviation that increases muscle tension in the neck and shoulders, potentially triggering migraine episodes. A study by Fernández-de-Las-Peñas et al. (2006) found that individuals with tension-type headaches exhibited a higher prevalence of FHP compared to asymptomatic controls, suggesting a link between this postural misalignment and headache disorders.

Further research indicates that neck pain is highly prevalent among individuals with primary headaches, including migraines. A cross-sectional study by Ashina et al. (2015) reported that 76.2% of participants with migraines experienced neck pain, compared to 56.7% of those without headaches. The study concluded that neck pain is significantly more common in individuals with migraines, highlighting the importance of addressing cervical musculoskeletal factors in headache management.

From my personal experience treating patients with migraines, I have consistently observed that they also suffer from tension headaches, which are often caused and triggered by poor posture, fibrotic tissue, and fascial restrictions. Poor neck posture, particularly forward head posture, can compress the **vertebral artery**, which supplies the brain with blood flow. This compression may reduce blood circulation to the brain, decreasing oxygen levels and triggering migraines. Many of my patients have reported significant improvement in their migraine symptoms after addressing these postural issues through manual therapy, postural correction exercises, and fascial release techniques.

Additionally, the American Migraine Foundation emphasizes that poor posture and prolonged periods of inactivity can contribute to increased migraine frequency. Maintaining a neutral head and neck position, ensuring proper back support, and avoiding prolonged static postures are recommended to mitigate these risks. Collectively, these findings underscore the significance of proper neck posture in the prevention and management of migraines.

Posture and Body Mechanics Training Videos Available Online.

Standing Posture
1. **Visualize a string**: Imagine a string coming out of the top of your head, pulling you upward towards the ceiling.
2. **Core engagement**: Keep your belly button sucked in.

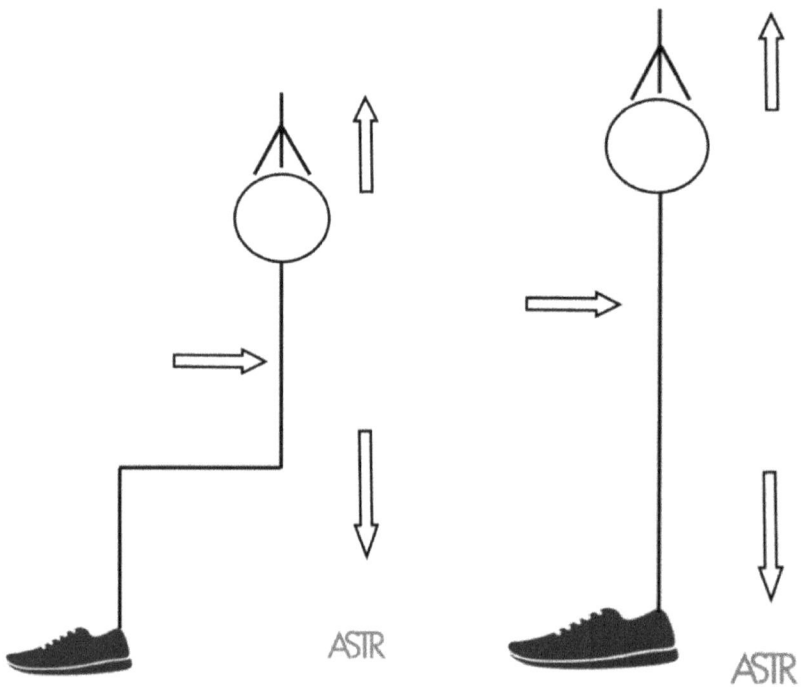

3. **Feet positioning**: Feet should be shoulder-width apart, with weight distributed through your heels.

Sitting Posture

1. **Visualize a string**: Imagine a string coming out of the top of your head, pulling you upward towards the ceiling.
2. **Engage your core**: Keep your belly button sucked in.
3. **Proper weight distribution**: Distribute your weight through your buttocks; keep your feet flat and shoulder-width apart.

Walking Posture

1. **Visualize a string**: Imagine a string coming out of the top of your head, pulling you upward towards the ceiling.
2. **Engage your core**: Suck your belly button in to stabilize your spine.

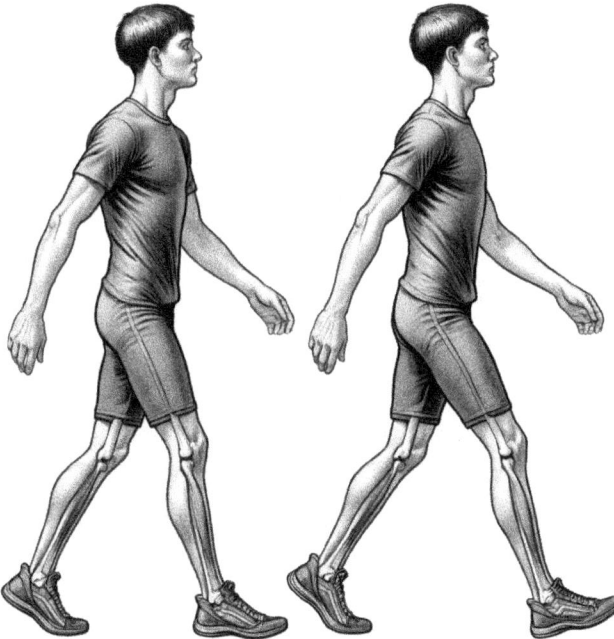

3. **Heel first**: Ensure your heel touches the ground first, then roll through to your toes.

General Tips

- **Start gradually**: Begin with short intervals, and progressively increase the duration you maintain these postures.

Posture

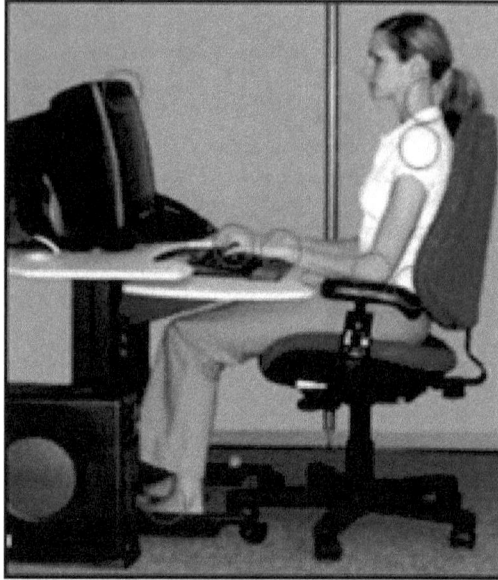

Image source: https://www.osha.gov/etools/computer-workstations

- **Be mindful**: Regularly check in with your body to ensure you're maintaining proper posture.
- **Create reminders**: Setting reminders can help you remember to adjust your posture throughout the day.

Correct Computer Posture

1. **Head and Neck Alignment**: Imagine a string pulling upward from the top of your head, keeping it level or slightly forward-facing and aligned with your torso. The neck should remain neutral, avoiding any tilting or twisting.
2. **Shoulder and Arm Position**: Shoulders should be relaxed, with upper arms hanging naturally at your sides. Elbows should be close to the body and bent at a 90-degree angle. Hands, wrists, and forearms should be straight, in-line, and roughly parallel to the floor, with forearms comfortably supported by armrests.
3. **Back Support**: Ensure your back is fully supported by the chair. Whether sitting upright or leaning back slightly, avoid twisting the back.
4. **Seat Positioning**: Thighs and hips should be supported by a well-padded seat, generally parallel to the floor. Knees should be at about the same height as the hips, with feet slightly forward.

5. **Foot Support**: Feet should rest fully on the floor. If the desk height is not adjustable and your feet do not comfortably reach the floor, use a footrest or a book to provide support.
6. **Monitor Setup**: Place the computer monitor directly in front of you, at eye level, to avoid straining your neck. The screen should be about an arm's length away, ensuring you do not have to tilt your head up, down, or sideways.

Additional Tips:
*   **Adjust your chair**: Make sure your chair height and backrest are adjustable to fit your body dimensions.
*   **Take breaks**: Regularly stand up, stretch, and walk around to relieve muscle tension and improve circulation.
*   **Monitor brightness and distance**: Adjust the brightness of your monitor to a comfortable level to reduce eye strain. Ensure the monitor is neither too close nor too far for comfortable viewing.
*   **Workspace layout**: Keep frequently used objects within easy reach to minimize reaching and twisting.

Implementing these practices can help reduce the risk of strain and discomfort. This contributes to a healthier, more productive work environment.

TV/Reading Posture
1. **Head and Neck Alignment**: Keep your head level or bent slightly forward, ensuring it remains in line with your torso. Your neck should be in a neutral position, not tilted to the side or excessively up or down.
2. **Eye Level**: Position your book or TV screen straight in front of you at eye level. This setup helps prevent neck strain by eliminating the need to look too far up, down, or to the side.
3. **Use a Reading Stand**: For reading, use a stand to hold your book. This reduces the strain on your arms and helps maintain a better neck posture.
4. **Shoulder Positioning**: Shoulders should be relaxed with upper arms hanging naturally at the sides. Avoid hunching or elevating your shoulders, which can lead to tension.
5. **Back Support**: Ensure your back is fully supported by the chair or sofa. Whether sitting upright or leaning back slightly, avoid twisting the back.

This supports the natural curve of your spine and reduces lower back strain.

6. **Arm and Hand Relaxation**:Use a reading stand or rest your forearm on a pillow so that your hands and arms can rest comfortably. This reduces the strain of holding up a book for long periods.

Additional Recommendations:
- **Lighting**: Ensure adequate lighting for reading to avoid eye strain. The light source should come from behind you, ideally over your shoulder, to illuminate the page or screen without causing glare.
- **Seating Choice**: Choose a comfortable chair or sofa that supports your posture with cushions if necessary. Consider a recliner or a chair with an adjustable back for added comfort.
- **Take Breaks**: Regularly change your position and take breaks to stretch and move around. This helps reduce muscle fatigue and stiffness from prolonged sitting.

Implementing these recommendations can greatly enhance your viewing and reading experience, promoting better posture and reducing the risk of discomfort or injury.

Correct Back Sleeping Posture
1. **Avoid Stomach Sleeping**: Sleeping on your stomach can put excessive strain on your neck and back. Instead, opt for back sleeping as it supports natural spinal alignment.
2. **Head and Neck Alignment**: Keep your head in a neutral position,

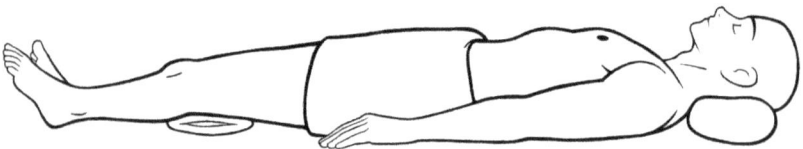

avoiding any flexion (tilting forward) or excessive side bending. Use a semi-firm contoured memory foam pillow that supports the natural curve of your neck.

3.   **Knee Support**: To maintain better spinal alignment and relieve pressure on your lower back, place a pillow under your knees. This helps flatten the lumbar region against the mattress and reduces stress on the spine.

Additional Tips:
- **Mattress Selection**: Choose a mattress that supports the contour of your spine. It should be firm enough to support your body but soft enough to allow for slight sinking of the heavier parts of your body.
- **Pillow Adjustments**: Ensure your pillow is not too high. It should just fill the space between your neck and the mattress to maintain proper alignment without lifting your head too high.
- **Relaxation Before Bed**: Engaging in relaxation techniques such as deep breathing before bed can help reduce muscle tension and promote better sleep.
- **Regular Review**: Evaluate your sleeping environment regularly to ensure it continues to meet your needs. This is especially important if you experience changes in health or comfort.

Implementing these practices not only improves your posture during sleep but can also enhance sleep quality. This helps prevent common discomforts associated with poor sleeping positions.

Correct Side Sleeping Posture
1.   **Avoid Stomach Sleeping**: Sleeping on your stomach is discouraged due to potential neck and back strain. Side sleeping is a healthier alternative that supports better spinal alignment.
2.   **Head and Neck Support**: Keep your head in a neutral position, avoiding any forward flexion or side bending. Use a semi-firm contoured memory foam pillow that adequately supports the natural curve of your neck. This aligns it with the rest of your spine.

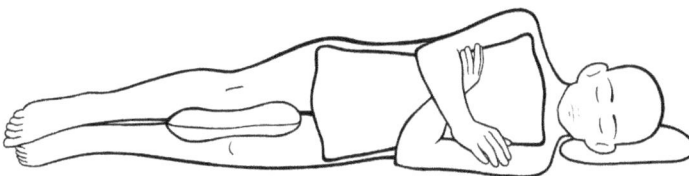

3. **Knee and Hip Alignment**: Place a pillow thick enough between your knees to ensure that your hips, knees, and ankles are aligned. This prevents the upper leg from pulling the spine out of alignment and reduces stress on the hips and lower back.

4. **Avoid Trunk Twisting**: Maintain your trunk in a straight alignment with your hips and shoulders stacked directly above each other. This prevents any twisting. Ensure your hips, knees, and ankles remain directly on top of each other.

5. **Use a Body Pillow**: A body pillow can be beneficial for side sleepers. It provides support for the arms and the entire body, helping to stabilize the trunk and prevent it from twisting during the night.

Additional Tips:

- **Pillow Adjustments**: Adjust the height and firmness of your pillow to ensure it fills the gap between your shoulder and the mattress. This helps maintain a straight neck and spine.
- **Mattress Firmness**: Choose a mattress that supports your body's weight while cushioning pressure points like hips and shoulders.
- **Regular Position Changes**: If feasible, alternate sides throughout the night to avoid overuse and strain on one side of your body.
- **Relaxation Techniques**: Engage in relaxing activities such as reading before bed to prepare your body for restful sleep.

Implementing these posture guidelines can greatly improve your sleep quality and contribute to overall spinal health.

Stress Management

The Link Between Stress and Migraines

Stress is one of the most commonly reported triggers for migraines, with approximately 70% of individuals with migraines identifying stress as a precipitating factor (American Migraine Foundation, 2020). Both major life events and daily stressors have been implicated in increasing migraine frequency and severity. Studies indicate that fluctuations in stress levels, rather than stress itself, may be a significant contributor to migraine onset. A study published in *Neurology* found that a reduction in perceived stress from one day to the next increased the likelihood of migraine onset within 6 to 18 hours, a phenomenon known as the "let-down" effect (Lipton et al., 2014). This suggests that the body's response to stress, rather than stress itself, plays a crucial role in triggering migraines.

The physiological mechanisms linking stress and migraines involve activation of the **hypothalamic-pituitary-adrenal (HPA) axis**, which regulates the body's stress response. During periods of acute stress, the body releases **cortisol** and other stress-related hormones, which have been found at elevated levels in individuals with migraines (Kim, 2024). Dysregulation of the HPA axis can contribute to migraine susceptibility by altering pain processing and increasing neuroinflammation (Borsook et al., 2012). Chronic stress has also been associated with increased central sensitization, a condition in which the nervous system becomes more sensitive to pain stimuli, thereby lowering the threshold for migraine attacks (Sauro & Becker, 2009).

Beyond physiological mechanisms, stress may also reduce the effectiveness of migraine treatments. Research indicates that individuals with higher levels of perceived stress often experience poorer responses to acute migraine therapies and greater migraine-related disability (Borsook et al., 2012). Interestingly, minor daily stressors, rather than major life events, appear to have a more substantial impact on migraine occurrence, emphasizing the importance of managing everyday stress in migraine prevention (Sauro & Becker, 2009).

Research studies showing that stress has consistently demonstrated its impact on various biological systems, potentially leading to a range of health issues. Here's a summary of how stress affects different parts of the body based on scientific studies:

1. Cardiovascular Effects: Stress may increase heart rate, blood pressure, and oxygen demand on the heart. It can also lead to vasoconstriction, increased blood lipids, and blood clotting issues, contributing to atherosclerosis and increased risk of heart attack and stroke.
2. Metabolic Effects: Stress can cause the liver to produce extra blood sugar (glucose), increasing the risk of developing type 2 diabetes
3. Gastrointestinal Effects: Stress can disrupt normal digestive function, leading to issues like heartburn, acid reflux, diarrhea, constipation, and stomach pain
4. Musculoskeletal Effects: Stress can cause muscles to tense up, leading to headaches, back pain, shoulder pain, and body aches.
5. Reproductive Effects: In men, stress can lower testosterone levels and interfere with sperm production and sexual function. In women, stress can disrupt the menstrual cycle.
6. Immune System Effects: Chronic stress can weaken the immune system, increasing susceptibility to infections.
7. Neurological/Psychological Effects: Stress can contribute to conditions like anxiety, depression, and insomnia. It can also impair cognitive function like memory and concentration.

Stress and muscle tension are closely related, and understanding this relationship can help in managing both effectively. Here's how stress leads to muscle tension and the potential long-term effects if it remains unaddressed:

Mechanisms of Muscle Tension Due to Stress

1. **Fight-or-Flight Response:** When you experience stress, your body's fight-or-flight response is triggered. This response prepares your body to either fight or flee from perceived threats. As part of this response, your muscles tense up, readying you for physical action. This was useful in ancient times when physical threats were common. However, in modern life, this response can be triggered by non-physical stresses like deadlines, traffic, or personal conflicts.
2. **Cortisol Release**: Stress stimulates the release of cortisol, a hormone that increases glucose in the bloodstream and enhances the brain's use of glucose. Cortisol also restricts functions that are non-essential in a

fight-or-flight situation, such as the immune response. High cortisol levels can lead to sustained muscle tension.

3. **Neuromuscular Reaction**: Stress affects the nervous system, which controls muscle activation. Under stress, the nervous system may keep muscles in a partly contracted state for prolonged periods.

Effects of Chronic Muscle Tension

1. **Pain and Discomfort**: Prolonged muscle tension can lead to muscle pain and discomfort, which might manifest as back pain, headaches, or neck pain. Tension-type headaches, one of the most common types of headaches, are directly linked to muscle tension in the neck and scalp.
2. **Reduced Mobility**: Over time, chronic muscle tension can reduce joint mobility. This stiffness can affect your posture and the way you move, potentially leading to mechanical imbalances and injury.
3. **Fibrotic tissue & Trigger Points**: Chronic tension can lead to the development of fibrotic tissue and trigger points—small knots that form in muscles and may cause pain in other parts of the body. These are often tender to the touch and can contribute to pain patterns seen in conditions like myofascial pain syndrome.
4. **Fatigue**: Muscles that are constantly under stress consume energy even when you're at rest. This can lead to muscle fatigue, which reduces your energy levels overall and can impact your physical performance.

Effective Strategies for Managing Stress

Managing stress effectively is crucial for maintaining both physical and mental health. Here are some practical tips for managing stress:

1. **Identify Stressors**: Keep a journal to identify the situations that create the most stress and how you respond to them. Noting patterns can help you find better coping strategies.
2. **Regular Physical Activity**: Exercise can help alleviate stress by producing endorphins (chemicals in the brain that act as natural painkillers) and improving your ability to sleep, which can reduce stress.
3. **Mindfulness and Meditation**: Techniques such as meditation, deep breathing exercises, and mindfulness can help melt away stress. Start

with just a few minutes a day and increase the duration as you feel more comfortable.

4. **Time Management**: Improve your time management skills to avoid feeling overwhelmed. Prioritize tasks, set boundaries, and break projects into manageable steps.
5. **Establish Boundaries**: In today's digital world, it's important to know when to turn off electronic devices. Set boundaries for work and social interactions to ensure personal time for relaxation.
6. **Nourish Your Body**: Eat a healthy diet. Well-nourished bodies are better prepared to cope with stress, so be mindful of what you eat.
7. **Sleep Adequately**: Ensure you get enough sleep. Lack of sleep is a significant contributor to stress. Most adults need 7-9 hours per night.
8. **Connect with Others**: Share your stress and concerns with friends or family members. Social connections can help you feel understood and supported.
9. **Practice Relaxation Techniques**: Engage in activities you enjoy, such as reading, yoga, or listening to music. Try relaxation techniques like progressive muscle relaxation or visualization.
10. **Seek Professional Help**: If your stress levels become too overwhelming, consider seeking professional help. Biopsychosocial therapist can help you learn how to manage stress effectively.

By incorporating these stress management tips into your life, you can find ways to reduce your stress levels and improve your overall well-being.

Meditation

Focused Breathing (Eyes Open or Closed)
- **Procedure**: Take a slow, deep breath in and out through your nose, filling your lungs with air.
- **Focus**: Concentrate on your breathing. If your mind wanders, gently redirect it to focus on your breathing.
- **Purpose**: This meditation breathing exercise can be used to help you go to sleep.
- **Session Duration**: 1 to 10 minutes, or as needed throughout the day.

Breathing Exercise I (Eyes Open)

- **Setting**: Can be done anywhere.
- **Procedure**:
  1. Take a slow, deep breath through your nose, filling your lungs with air.
  2. Hold your breath for 5 to 15 seconds.
  3. Exhale slowly through your nose.
  4. Repeat this process 20 times per session.
- **Focus**: Concentrate on your breathing and redirect your focus if your mind wanders.
- **Frequency**: Perform 4-5 sessions per day.

Breathing Exercise II (Eyes Closed)
- **Setting**: Perform this exercise in a quiet room.
- **Position**: Sit in a comfortable chair with back support, rest your arms on a pillow in your lap, and keep your feet flat on the floor (shoulder width apart).
- **Procedure**:
  1. Take a slow, deep breath in through your nose.
  2. Hold your breath for 5 to 15 seconds.
  3. Exhale slowly through your nose.
  4. Repeat this process 20 times per session.
- **Focus**: Concentrate on your breathing and redirect your focus if your mind wanders.
- **Frequency**: Perform 4-5 sessions per day.

Breathing Exercise III (Eyes Closed)
- **Setting**: Perform this exercise in a quiet room.
- **Position**: Sit in a comfortable chair with back support, rest your arms on a pillow in your lap, and keep your feet flat on the floor (shoulder width apart).
- **Procedure**:
  1. Take a slow, deep breath in through your nose.
  2. Hold your breath for 5 to 15 seconds.
  3. Exhale slowly through your mouth while making a vibration sound.
  4. Repeat this process 40 times per session.

- **Focus**: Concentrate on your breathing and redirect your focus if your mind wanders.
- **Frequency**: Perform 2-3 sessions per day.

Conclusion

Managing stress is an essential part of reducing the frequency and intensity of migraines. Chronic stress activates the body's fight or flight response, which can lead to inflammation, muscle tension, hormonal disruption, and neurological overstimulation, key factors that can trigger or worsen migraines. While this chapter provides effective tools for managing everyday stress, it is important to recognize that deeper emotional struggles such as anxiety, depression, and post-traumatic stress disorder (PTSD) require more comprehensive support.

If you are dealing with chronic anxiety, emotional overwhelm, or unresolved trauma, I encourage you to explore my companion book *Beating Anxiety and Depression: 14 Natural Secrets to a Happier Life*. This book offers a step-by-step natural approach to emotional healing backed by research and clinical experience. It addresses the biological, psychological, and lifestyle factors that contribute to mental health struggles and provides actionable strategies to restore emotional balance.

Due to the complexity of mental health conditions, it is difficult to do justice to this topic in just one chapter. That is why *Beating Anxiety and Depression* was created as a complete resource for those seeking long-term relief from anxiety, depression, and PTSD. If emotional stress plays a role in your migraines or if you are simply looking to improve your mental well-being, this book is a powerful next step on your healing journey.

BEATING
ANXIETY
&
DEPRESSION

BONUS VIDEOS

14 NATURAL SECRETS TO A HAPPIER LIFE

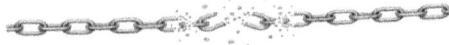

- Conquer Anxiety & Depression Naturally
- Heal the Root Causes & Reclaim Your Life
- Created by a Doctor Who Conquered PTSD & Depression
- Science-Based Strategies for Lasting Change

Dr. Joseph Jacobs, DPT, ACN

Fibrotic Tissue

Do you tend to slouch or hunch forward when using your phone or computer? Believe it or not, poor posture can cause fibrotic tissue (scar tissue) to build up in the neck and shoulders. If possible, place your hand on the back of your shoulder, close to your neck, and press firmly. If you notice a hard knot, it's possible that you have fibrotic tissue (scar tissue) as a result of poor posture. Since we cannot visually see internal fibrotic tissue, it is often overlooked and ignored. Our muscles should act like a rubber band, contracting and relaxing to encourage a full range of motion in the joint. However, fibrotic tissue acts like a knot in the rubber band, limiting its full range of motion. Patients with fibrotic tissue may experience pain and decreased range of motion. If left untreated, this condition can lead to nerve damage, chronic pain, and may even require surgery.

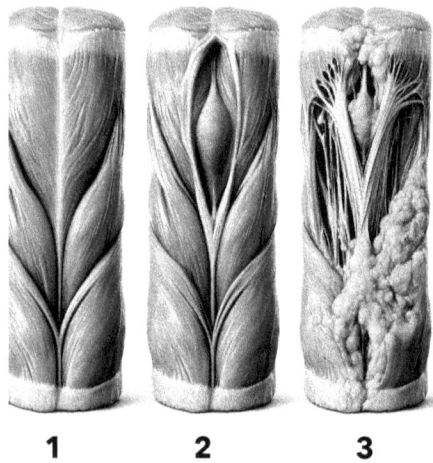

1 **2** **3**

Image Explanation

1. **Healthy, intact muscle:** An illustration showing the muscle fibers in their natural, unbroken state.
2. **Muscle with tear:** An illustration depicting a clear gap in the tissue where the muscle fibers are disrupted and separated.
3. **Muscle with fibrotic tissue:** An illustration of a muscle with a tear and dense, scar-like fibrotic tissue contrasting with the normal muscle fibers.

Fibrotic tissue, characterized by the excessive accumulation of extracellular matrix components leading to tissue stiffness and scarring, has been implicated in various musculoskeletal disorders. While direct research linking fibrotic tissue to migraines is limited, related studies suggest potential mechanisms through which fibrosis may contribute to migraine pathophysiology.

One pertinent area of investigation is the role of neurogenic inflammation in migraine development. Neurogenic inflammation involves the release of neuropeptides, such as substance P and calcitonin gene-related peptide (CGRP), from sensory nerve endings, leading to vasodilation and increased vascular permeability. This process can result in tissue edema and may promote fibrotic changes in the affected tissues. A review by Edvinsson and Uddman (2005) highlighted the involvement of neuropeptides in migraine pathophysiology, suggesting that their release contributes to the inflammatory processes associated with migraine attacks.

Additionally, the concept of central sensitization, a condition where the central nervous system becomes hypersensitive to stimuli, is relevant. Central sensitization is a key feature in chronic migraine sufferers and is associated with increased responsiveness to pain. This heightened sensitivity can lead to alterations in pain perception and may be linked to structural changes in neural tissues, potentially involving fibrotic processes. A study by Burstein et al. (2015) discussed the role of central sensitization in migraine chronification, indicating that persistent activation of pain pathways can lead to long-term changes in the brain's structure and function.

Furthermore, fibrotic changes in cervical musculature and connective tissues could contribute to myofascial pain syndromes, which are often comorbid with migraines. Restricted mobility and increased tissue stiffness resulting from fibrosis may exacerbate musculoskeletal strain, potentially triggering migraine episodes. While direct evidence is scarce, understanding the interplay between fibrotic tissue changes and migraine pathophysiology could inform more comprehensive treatment approaches.

In my clinical experience, patients with migraines often present with increased tissue stiffness and reduced flexibility in the cervical and cranial musculature. Implementing manual therapies aimed at reducing tissue fibrosis, such as myofascial release and fibrotic tissue release, has led to notable improvements in headache frequency, intensity, and overall quality of life.

Collectively, these insights suggest that fibrotic tissue changes may play a role in migraine pathogenesis, particularly through mechanisms involving neurogenic inflammation and central sensitization. Addressing fibrotic tissue restrictions through targeted therapeutic interventions may offer additional avenues for managing migraine symptoms.

Fibroblasts

Fibroblasts are a type of cell that are essential for wound healing and play a critical role in the maintenance and repair of connective tissues throughout the body. They are the most common cells of connective tissue in animals. They are typically active during the proliferation phase of the healing process. Fibroblasts are a type of cell most commonly found within connective tissues in animals. They play a crucial role in the structural framework of tissues by producing and maintaining the extracellular matrix, which is the complex scaffold of proteins and other substances that support cells. Fibroblasts are responsible for producing key components of this matrix, including collagen, fibronectin, and elastin, which help provide structural integrity and elasticity to tissues.

During wound healing or in response to injury, fibroblasts are activated and multiply. They are crucial in the healing process as they migrate to the site of injury, where they produce collagen and other extracellular matrix components to form fibrotic tissue and repair the damaged tissue. In pathological conditions, fibroblasts can become overly active. This leads to excessive deposition of connective and fibrotic tissue, which can disrupt normal tissue architecture and function.

Here are some key functions and characteristics of fibroblasts:
1. **Tissue Repair and Maintenance**: Fibroblasts produce and secrete collagen and other extracellular matrix proteins that form the structural framework for tissues such as skin, tendons, and ligaments.

2. **Wound Healing**: During the process of wound healing, fibroblasts are activated and migrate to the site of injury. They proliferate and produce collagen and other fibers, which help in closing and healing the wound.
3. **Fibrotic Tissue Formation**: In the proliferation stages of wound healing, fibroblasts help in the formation of fibrotic tissue by depositing excess collagen. This can sometimes lead to the overproduction of fibrosis.
4. **Role in Diseases**: Abnormal function and activation of fibroblasts can contribute to a variety of pathological conditions, including fibrosis (excessive fibrous connective tissue formation) and autoimmune diseases such as rheumatoid arthritis and systemic sclerosis.

Fibroblasts can also differentiate into myofibroblasts, especially during wound healing, which possess contractile capabilities similar to muscle cells, aiding in the contraction of the wound.

Fibrosis

Fibrosis is defined by the overgrowth, hardening, and/or scarring of various tissues and is attributed to the excess deposition of extracellular matrix components, including collagen. Fibrosis characterizes a pathological state of excessive tissue repair where there is an overgrowth, hardening, and scarring of tissue primarily due to the excessive deposition of extracellular matrix components such as collagen. This process can affect virtually any tissue in the body, leading to significant organ dysfunction depending on the site and severity of the fibrotic response.

Fibrosis often results from chronic inflammatory reactions triggered by a variety of stimuli. These can include:

- **Poor posture and body mechanics:** This is considered a repetitive strain injury due to prolonged poor posture and body mechanics, which cause muscle strain and tendon sprains. This strain leads to inflammation, and eventually, the body builds excessive fibrotic tissue.
- **Persistent infections:** Where ongoing microbial presence provokes a sustained immune response.
- **Autoimmune reactions:** Where the body's immune system mistakenly attacks its own tissues.
- **Allergic responses:** Which can cause chronic inflammation due to repeated exposure to allergens.

- **Chemical insults:** Such as exposure to toxins or irritants that cause tissue damage and subsequent fibrotic repair.
- **Radiation:** Which can damage cells and extracellular matrix, leading to scarring and fibrosis.
- **Physical tissue injury:** From events like trauma or surgery, which initiates the healing process that can sometimes lead to excessive scar tissue formation if the healing process is dysregulated.

The fibrotic process involves complex signaling pathways and cellular interactions, primarily involving fibroblasts, as mentioned earlier. These fibroblasts play a key role in synthesizing and remodeling the extracellular matrix during both normal tissue repair and pathological fibrosis.

Understanding the function of fibroblasts and regulating their activity can be crucial for managing and treating various conditions involving tissue repair and fibrosis. Fibrotic tissue, often known as scar tissue, is a type of connective tissue that forms during the wound healing process, particularly during the proliferation stage. It mainly consists of collagen, a protein that provides structural strength. While essential for repairing damaged areas, excessive fibrotic tissue can lead to muscle or joint pain and restricted range of motion.

Characteristics of Fibrotic Tissue
1. **Composition**: Fibrotic tissue has a higher density of collagen fibers compared to normal tissue. These fibers are often more disorganized and aligned differently than in the original tissue, which can affect the flexibility and functionality of the area.
2. **Elasticity**: Scar tissue is less elastic and more fibrous than the original tissue. This can lead to stiffness and restricted movement, especially if the fibrosis occurs near joints.
3. **Vascularity**: Fibrotic tissue typically has fewer blood vessels than the original tissue, making it appear paler and potentially leading to a slower metabolic rate in that area.
4. **Sensory Nerves**: fibrotic tissue may have fewer sensory nerves, which can result in areas of numbness or altered sensation.

Causes of Fibrosis
Fibrosis can result from a variety of conditions and scenarios, including:

- **Injury:** Following trauma or surgery, fibrotic tissue develops as part of the natural healing process to close the wound site. If the wound site remains open, it is susceptible to infection. Fibrotic tissues are crucial for our survival. However, the problem arises when excessive fibrotic tissue forms, which can compress blood vessels and nerves, limit range of motion, and cause pain.
- **Chronic Inflammation**: Diseases that cause long-term inflammation can lead to excessive fibrotic tissue formation. This is seen in conditions such as rheumatoid arthritis, osteoarthritis, fibromyalgia, ankylosing spondylitis, psoriatic arthritis, systemic lupus erythematosus, tendonitis, bursitis, and various autoimmune diseases.
- **Repeated Injury or Irritation**: Areas of the body that undergo repeated stress or injury can become chronically inflamed and subsequently fibrotic.
- **Disease Processes**: Certain diseases can promote fibrosis. These include conditions such as liver cirrhosis from chronic hepatitis or liver damage, pulmonary fibrosis in the lungs, and systemic diseases like scleroderma, which affects connective tissue.
- **Stretching:** Frequent and intense stretching can lead to inflammation and overstimulation of fibroblasts. This can result in increased collagen production and potentially lead to excessive fibrotic tissue formation within the tendons.
- **Poor posture and body mechanics:** This is considered a repetitive strain injury due to prolonged poor posture and body mechanics, which cause muscle strain and tendon sprains. This strain leads to inflammation, and eventually, the body builds excessive fibrotic tissue.

Impact of Fibrotic Tissue

Excessive fibrotic tissue in the body can have a range of detrimental effects, impacting various organs and systems. Fibrosis is essentially the thickening and scarring of connective tissue, usually resulting from a healing process in response to injury or long-term inflammation. Here are some key impacts of excessive fibrotic tissue:

- **Nerve damage:** If excessive fibrotic tissue compresses nerve cells, it could cause numbness, tingling sensations, or permanent nerve damage, resulting in loss of function and sensation. This can occur in conditions such as sciatica, carpal tunnel syndrome, and others.

- **Chronic Pain:** Fibrosis can lead to chronic pain, especially when it affects muscles, joints, or tissues involved in movement. Conditions such as Dupuytren's contracture, back pain, neck pain, sciatica, carpal tunnel syndrome, bursitis, tendonitis, plantar fasciitis, frozen shoulder, tension headaches, and trigger finger are examples where fibrosis can significantly contribute to discomfort and mobility issues.
- **Mobility Issues**: In muscles, tendons, and ligaments, fibrosis can restrict movement, leading to stiffness and pain. Typically, our muscles behave like a rubber band, stretching and elongating as they contract and relax. However, when fibrotic tissue is present in the muscle, it acts like a knot that limits muscle contraction, reduces range of motion, and causes pain.
- **Reduced Functionality**: Fibrotic tissue is less flexible than normal tissue, which can lead to impaired function of the affected organ or area. For example, in the lungs (as in pulmonary fibrosis), this can lead to difficulty breathing and decreased oxygen intake.
- **Organ Dysfunction**: In organs like the liver (cirrhosis), heart (cardiac fibrosis), and kidneys (renal fibrosis), excessive fibrotic tissue can disrupt normal function. This can result in a significant decrease in the organ's ability to perform its essential tasks, such as filtering blood, pumping blood, or metabolizing substances.
- **Increased Risk of Complications**: Fibrotic changes can increase the risk of further complications. For instance, liver cirrhosis, which involves fibrosis or scarring of the liver, can lead to complications such as portal hypertension and visceral bleeding.
- **Impaired Healing and Regeneration**: Excessive fibrosis can interfere with the normal healing process, as scar tissue can replace normal, healthy tissue, leading to prolonged or incomplete recovery.
- **Restricted Movement**: In cases where fibrosis affects the skin, muscles, or connective tissues (such as in scleroderma or after severe burns), it can lead to reduced mobility due to stiff and tightened tissues.
- **Aesthetic Concerns**: On the skin, fibrotic tissue can cause cosmetic concerns, especially if the scarring is extensive or occurs in highly visible areas.

Ineffective Methods for Breaking Down Fibrotic Tissue

Fibrotic tissue, due to its thickness and hardness, requires firm mechanical force to break down. An understanding of the physiology of fibrosis shows that certain approaches are ineffective for breaking down fibrotic tissue. These include massage, foam rollers, manual therapy, Gua Sha, instrument-assisted soft tissue mobilization, stretching, and exercises.

1. **Foam rollers:** These approaches typically provide only superficial pressure on the tissue. In many cases, fibrotic tissue is located deep within muscles, such as in the hamstrings, quadriceps, and gluteus muscles, where it can be up to 2 inches deep. This renders foam rollers ineffective for reaching and treating these areas.
2. **Deep tissue massage:** Involves the therapist using their hands, knuckles, and/or elbows to reach deeper layers of muscle. However, due to the width and diameter of the therapist's knuckles and elbows, it is difficult to penetrate deep tissues and provide consistent forces necessary to break down deep fibrotic tissue
3. **Manual therapy:** Similar to massage, manual therapy often involves using the knuckles, elbows, or hands to reach deeper tissues. However, the relatively large diameter of the therapist's hands and elbows may limit their ability to penetrate deeply enough to effect physiological changes in fibrotic tissues located deep within muscles.
4. **Exercises and Stretching:** Do not exert sufficient mechanical force on fibrotic tissue to break it down; they simply cause movement in the muscle.
5. **Myofascial release:** Involves applying gentle, sustained pressure to the superficial connective tissue, which may not exert enough mechanical force to break down scar tissue or reach deeply enough to affect deep fibrosis.
6. **Gua Sha and Instrument-Assisted Soft Tissue Mobilization:** These techniques involve tools that might resemble rods or a butter knife, used to apply horizontal superficial force on the skin. Like manual therapy, they fail to penetrate deeply enough to alter fibrotic tissue effectively. This is like trying to unscrew a deep-set screw in a car with a screwdriver that is too short; it simply cannot reach deep enough to be effective.

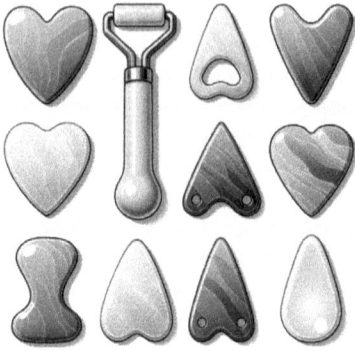

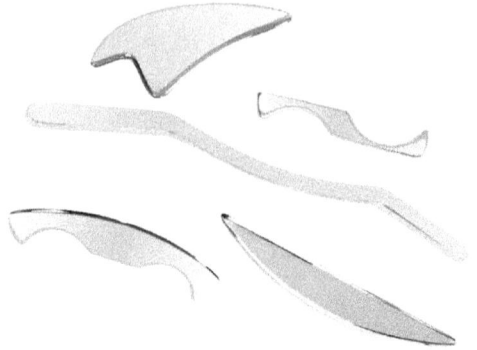

Instrument Assisted Soft Tissue Mobilization (IASTM)

Gua Sha

The Solution

Analyzing and testing current approaches that claim to break down fibrotic tissue led me to realize that it is physiologically impossible to effectively target both superficial and deep fibrotic tissue with these methods. This realization was the turning point that inspired the invention of ergonomically designed ASTR instruments. These instruments are specifically created to address both superficial and deep fibrotic tissue, capable of penetrating up to 2 inches deep to break down adhesions.

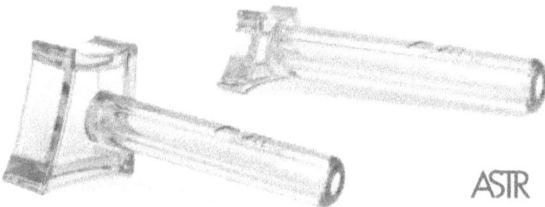

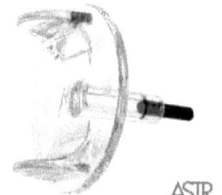

Conclusion

In chronic migraine conditions, the affected areas of the body often become trapped in a persistent cycle of inflammation and tissue proliferation, preventing proper healing. This ongoing cycle leads to heightened inflammation, fibrosis, muscle spasms, and severe fascial restrictions, which contribute to the intensity and frequency of migraines. Nutritional deficiencies in essential vitamins and minerals can further hinder the body's ability to progress to the final stage of healing, keeping it locked in this disruptive pattern. Additionally, excessive fibrosis and fascial tightness can worsen the condition, making it even more difficult to break free from the cycle of chronic migraines.

Fascial Restrictions

Myofascial restrictions, particularly the presence of myofascial trigger points (MTrPs), have been implicated in the pathophysiology of migraines. MTrPs are hyperirritable spots within taut bands of skeletal muscle fibers that can elicit local and referred pain upon palpation. Research indicates a high prevalence of active MTrPs in migraine patients, especially in the temporal, suboccipital, and sternocleidomastoid muscles. A recent study found that 93% of individuals with migraines had active MTrPs in these regions, suggesting a significant association between myofascial dysfunction and migraine occurrence.

The presence of MTrPs may contribute to migraines by increasing pericranial muscle tenderness and sensitizing central pain pathways. A study by Fernández-de-Las-Peñas et al. (2006) reported that patients with unilateral migraines exhibited a higher prevalence of MTrPs in the upper trapezius, sternocleidomastoid, and temporalis muscles compared to healthy controls. This finding suggests that MTrPs in these muscles may play a role in migraine pathogenesis.

Interventions targeting myofascial restrictions have shown promise in alleviating migraine symptoms. A randomized controlled trial investigated the effects of myofascial release on migraine patients. The study found significant reductions in pain intensity and neck disability, as well as increased cervical range of motion in the treatment group compared to controls. These results indicate that addressing myofascial dysfunction can be an effective component of migraine management.

Furthermore, a meta-analysis assessing the efficacy of myofascial release (MFR) interventions concluded that MFR significantly alleviates pain and disability in patients with tension-type and cervicogenic headaches. While the results for migraine were inconsistent, the analysis suggests potential benefits of MFR in reducing headache-related symptoms.

In my clinical experience, patients with migraines often present with palpable myofascial restrictions and active MTrPs in the cervical and cranial musculature. Implementing manual therapies aimed at releasing these restrictions, such as myofascial release has led to notable improvements in headache frequency, intensity, and overall quality of life.

Collectively, these findings underscore the importance of evaluating and addressing myofascial dysfunction in individuals suffering from migraines. Incorporating myofascial release techniques into a comprehensive treatment plan may offer significant benefits in reducing migraine-related pain and disability.

The fascial system, an integral component of the body's connective tissue network, plays a crucial role in supporting and connecting all bodily structures. Here's a comprehensive overview of the fascial system:

What is Fascia?

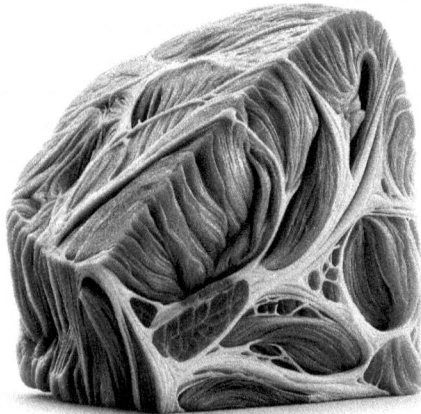

The white filaments in the meat are the fascia layers

Next time you buy meat, look for the white filaments in it; those are the fascia layers. Fascia is a dense, tough tissue that extends throughout the body in a three-dimensional web from head to toe. It surrounds and interpenetrates every muscle, bone, nerve, blood vessel, and organ. Fascia is primarily made up of collagen fibers, which provide it with both flexibility and strength. Fascia is a complex network of connective tissue that extends throughout the body and plays a crucial role in supporting and protecting bodily structures.

Key Attributes of the Fascial System

The fascia system, a continuous network of connective tissue that envelops and interconnects every structure in the body, plays a critical role in maintaining overall health and physical integrity. Here are the key attributes of the fascial system:

1. Ubiquity and Continuity

- Fascia is present throughout the entire body. It wraps around and interconnects muscles, bones, organs, nerves, and blood vessels, forming a seamless web that extends from head to toe. This continuity is crucial for the integration and coordination of bodily structures and functions.

2. Structural Support and Protection

- Fascia provides a framework that supports the body's structures. It helps maintain the position of organs, enables the transmission of muscular force, and protects internal structures from physical trauma.

3. Flexibility and Elasticity

- Despite its strength, fascia is also highly flexible and elastic. This allows it to stretch and move without restriction, accommodating movements of muscles and joints while returning to its original shape.

4. Sensory Role

- Fascia is richly innervated with nerve endings, making it an important sensory organ. These nerves are responsible for proprioception (the sense of body position and movement) and the perception of pain. This sensory role is essential for maintaining posture and physical coordination.

5. Fluid Transport

- The fascial network plays a role in the circulation of fluids throughout the body, including blood and lymphatic fluid. It facilitates the transport of nutrients and waste products to and from cells.

6. Metabolic Function

- Fascia can store energy in the form of fat and water, and it also provides pathways for inflammation and healing. The extracellular matrix within the fascia contains cells that can respond to and influence metabolic processes.

7. Adaptability

- Fascia is highly adaptable and responsive to physical and emotional stimuli. Chronic stress, injury, or poor postural habits can lead to changes in the fascial structures, sometimes leading to restrictions and pain.

8. Pathway for Force Transmission

- Fascia transmits mechanical tension generated by muscle activity or external forces across the body. This distribution of force helps in reducing local stress on muscles and joints and enhances overall movement efficiency.

9. Compartmentalization

- Through deeper layers, such as the deep fascia, it compartmentalizes sections of the body, segregating groups of muscles and other structures into functional units. This compartmentalization aids in organizing the body architecturally and facilitates effective movement and function.

These attributes illustrate why the fascial system is integral not only to movement and stability but also to the general health and well-being of the body. Understanding and addressing fascial health is crucial in sports, rehabilitation, and general physical maintenance.

Layers of the Fascial System

There are several distinct layers of fascia, each with its specific function and characteristics. Understanding these layers helps in appreciating the complexity of human anatomy and the integration of bodily functions. Here's a detailed explanation of the different fascia layers:

1. **Superficial Fascia (Subcutaneous Tissue)**
   - **Location**: The superficial fascia layer is like a Spider-Man suit covering the whole body. Just below the skin, above the deeper layers of fascia.This layer separates the skin from the musculoskeletal system, allowing for normal sliding between the muscles and skin.
   - **Composition**: Consists of loose connective tissue and fat. This layer varies in thickness across different parts of the body and from person to person. Many nerve fibers are observed, and in some regions, the superficial fascia splits, forming specialized compartments. The collagen fibers are arranged irregularly. It consists of different layers that can slide over one another. The superficial fascia layer consists of two to three layers on top of each other

- **Functions**: Acts as a water storage medium, provides insulation and padding, and allows the skin to move freely over underlying structures. It also serves as a conduit for nerves and blood vessels as they pass to and from the skin.

2. **Deep Fascia**
   - **Location**: Surrounds and infuses with muscles, bones, nerves, and blood vessels to the level of the dermis.
   - **Composition**: Denser than superficial fascia, this layer is made of tightly packed collagen fibers running in a parallel arrangement. It forms a fibrous sheath that encloses muscles and divides them into groups. Each

Musclar Fascia Layers

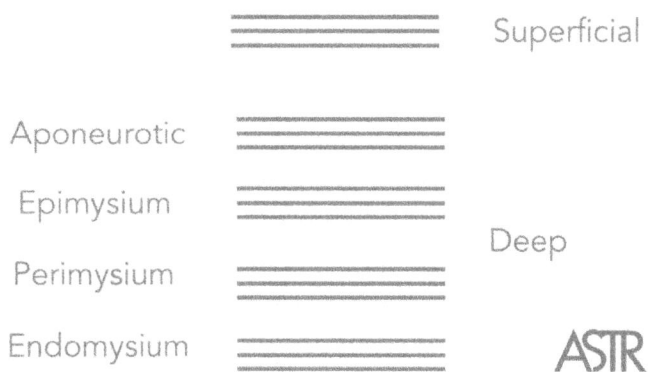

Superficial

Aponeurotic

Epimysium

Perimysium   Deep

Endomysium   ASTR

subdivision of the deep fascia layer consists of two to three layers on top of each other.
   - **Functions**: Provides an extensive area for muscle attachment, enhances force transmission across muscles, and maintains structural integrity. The deep fascia also separates different functional areas of muscles, allowing them to operate independently.

Division of Deep Fascia:

- **Aponeurotic Fascia:** Surrounds groups of muscles. It consists of 2 or 3 layers of unidirectional collagen fibers, with each layer separated by loose connective tissue. Composed of 80% collagen fibers and only 1% elastic fibers. This fascia helps keep a group of muscles in place or serves as the insertion point for a broad muscle.
- **Epimysial Fascia:** Surrounds the entire muscle. It is formed of type I and III collagen and is specific to each muscle. It contains approximately 15% elastic fibers. The epimysium is free to glide due to being separated from the aponeurotic fascia by an external layer of loose connective tissue. It is thinner than the aponeurotic fascia and is also separated from the perimysial fascia by an internal layer of loose connective tissue. Multiple septa detach from the epimysium and insert into both the overlying aponeurotic fascia and the underlying perimysial fascia.
- **Perimysial Fascia:** Surrounds bundles of muscle fibers within a muscle. It consists of connective tissue that penetrates the muscle to support and separate muscle fiber bundles (fascicles). This fascia provides the pathway for nerves and blood vessels to reach individual muscle fibers.
- **Endomysial Fascia:** Surrounds individual muscle fibers. It is a thin layer of connective tissue that supports capillaries and nerve fibers. The endomysium plays a crucial role in the transfer of force from the muscle fibers to the tendons.

3. **Visceral Fascia (Subserous Fascia)**
    - **Location**: Surrounds organs within the cavities of the body, such as the thoracic and abdominal cavities.
    - **Composition**: Thinner and more delicate than deep fascia, and often contains a larger amount of elastic fibers to accommodate the movement and expansion of organs.
    - **Functions**: The fascia holds organs in place and provides them with structural support. It also creates compartments within the body that can help limit the spread of infections or malignancies.

    Each layer of fascia is integral to the functional architecture of the body, providing both structural support and flexibility. Problems in any layer of the fascia can lead to pain, reduced function, and mobility issues, highlighting the importance of this connective tissue system in overall health and well-being.

Functions of the Fascial System

The fascial system has several crucial functions:
1. **Support and Structure**: Fascia provides a supportive and stabilizing framework for all body structures. It holds organs in place and ensures that muscles and other structures maintain their proper alignment.
2. **Force Transmission**: Through its tensile strength and structural continuity, fascia transmits mechanical loads and muscle forces efficiently across the body. This helps in maintaining balance and coordination during movement.
3. **Protection**: Fascia acts as a protective layer over muscles and organs, cushioning them and reducing the impact of external forces.
4. **Separation and Compartmentalization**: By forming natural divisions between muscles and organs, fascia allows different body structures to slide smoothly over each other, facilitating efficient movement.

Fascial restrictions

Fascia restrictions, often simply referred to as fascial restrictions, occur when the fascia, the connective tissue that surrounds and supports all structures within the body, becomes tight, stiff, or forms adhesions. These restrictions can significantly impact the body's mobility, flexibility, and function. Here's an in-depth look at fascia restrictions:

Fascial restrictions refer to the tightening or stiffening of the fascia, the connective tissue that surrounds and supports muscles, bones, nerves, and organs throughout the body. Fascia is supposed to be flexible and able to stretch as you move. However, due to various factors such as injury, surgery, inflammation, poor posture, or lack of activity, the fascia can become restricted. When fascial restrictions occur, they can limit mobility and cause pain, discomfort, or decreased range of motion. These restrictions can have a cascading effect on the body, potentially affecting overall biomechanical efficiency and leading to compensations in movement, which in turn might cause further discomfort or injury.

Fascia Adhesion

Fascia adhesion occurs when the fascia, a thin layer of connective tissue that surrounds muscles, organs, and other structures, sticks to itself or to other tissues. This can restrict movement and cause pain.

Fascia Fibrosis

Fascia fibrosis is the thickening and stiffening of the fascia due to excessive collagen deposition, often as a response to chronic inflammation or injury. This condition is more severe than simple adhesions and can significantly impair function.

Causes of Fascia Restrictions
Fascia restrictions can arise from a variety of factors:
- **Injury**: Trauma from accidents or surgeries can lead to inflammation and subsequent fibrosis (scar tissue), which restricts the normal elasticity of fascia.
- **Repetitive Stress**: Repetitive activities or overuse injuries can lead to chronic inflammation and fibrotic changes in the fascia.
- **Poor Posture**: Prolonged poor posture can cause the fascia to adapt in maladaptive ways, leading to tension and restrictions.
- **Inactivity**: Lack of movement can cause fascia to become dehydrated and less pliable, making it prone to stiffness and adhesions.
- **Inflammatory Responses**: Systemic inflammation, as seen in various autoimmune disorders, can also affect the fascial system, making it less flexible.

Symptoms of Fascia Restrictions
The presence of fascial restrictions can manifest in various symptoms:
- **Reduced Mobility**: Stiffness and limited range of motion in joints.
- **Pain**: Chronic pain is often described as a deep, aching, or band-like pain that may increase with movement or touch.
- **Tension**: A feeling of tightness in the muscles and surrounding areas.
- **Sensory Changes**: Some individuals might experience tingling or numbness due to the pressure on nerves by tight fascia.
- **Misalignment**: Fascial restrictions can pull the body out of alignment, affecting posture and leading to compensatory patterns elsewhere in the body.

Ineffective Methods for Releasing Fascial Restrictions

The fascia system is so complex that it requires targeted tools to release each restricted layer. Random hand movements without gripping the fascia layer will not mobilize it to release the adhesions that cause the layers to stick together and prevent them from gliding freely on top of each other. An understanding of the physiology of the fascia system shows that certain approaches are ineffective for releasing it, including massage, foam rollers, manual therapy, Gua Sha, instrument-assisted soft tissue mobilization, stretching, and exercises.

1. **Foam rollers:** Typically, they provide only superficial pressure on the tissue. Gliding the foam roller over just the superficial layer will not release the adhesions, and the foam roller will not apply enough deep pressure to release the epimysium, perimysium, and endomysium layers.
2. **Deep tissue massage:** Involves the therapist using their hands, knuckles, and/or elbows to reach deeper layers of muscle. However, due to the width and diameter of the therapist's knuckles and elbows, it is difficult to penetrate deep tissues and provide the consistent gripping forces necessary to release deep fascia adhesions.
3. **Manual therapy:** Similar to massage, it often involves using the knuckles, elbows, or hands to reach deeper tissues. However, the relatively large diameter of the therapist's hands and elbows may limit their ability to penetrate deeply enough to effect physiological changes in fascia layers located deep within muscles. Additionally, it is very difficult for the hand to grip deep fascia layers to release them.
4. **Exercises and stretching:** Do not exert sufficient mechanical force on fascia layers to cause adhesion release; they simply cause movement in the muscle.
5. **Myofascial release:** This involves applying gentle, sustained pressure to the superficial connective tissue, which addresses the superficial fascia layer but does not go deep enough to release the aponeurotic, epimysium, perimysium, and endomysium fascia layers.
6. **Gua Sha and Instrument-Assisted Soft Tissue Mobilization:** These techniques involve tools that might resemble rods or a butter knife, used to apply horizontal superficial force on the skin. Like manual therapy, they fail to penetrate deeply enough to alter the fascia system and are unable to grip

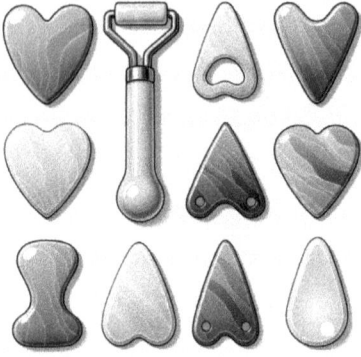

Gua Sha

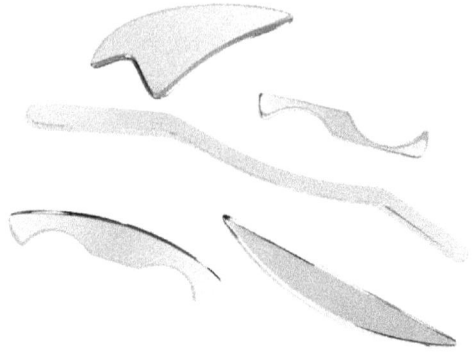

Instrument Assisted Soft Tissue Mobilization (IASTM)

the fascia layers to release them. This is like trying to unscrew a deep-set screw in a car with a screwdriver that is too short; it simply cannot reach deep enough to be effective.

The Solution

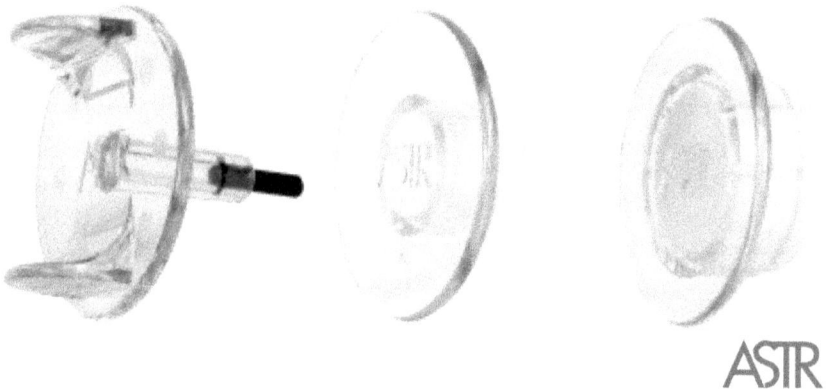

ASTR

Analyzing and testing current approaches that claim to provide myofascial release led me to realize that it is physiologically impossible to effectively target both superficial and deep fascia layers with these methods. This realization was the turning point that inspired the invention of ergonomically designed ASTR instruments. These instruments are specifically created to address superficial fascia, aponeurotic fascia, epimysium, perimysium, and endomysium layers. They are capable of penetrating up to 2 inches deep to release the epimysium, perimysium, and endomysium.

Conclusion

In chronic migraine conditions, the body often becomes trapped in a continuous cycle of inflammation and tissue proliferation, preventing proper healing. This ongoing process leads to widespread inflammation, fibrosis, muscle spasms, and severe fascial restrictions, all of which contribute to the persistence and intensity of migraines. Deficiencies in essential vitamins and minerals can further disrupt the body's ability to progress to the final stage of healing, keeping it locked in this dysfunctional pattern. Additionally, excessive fibrosis and fascial tension can amplify the condition, making it even more difficult to break free from the cycle of chronic migraines.

This persistent cycle highlights the limitations of the biomedical model in effectively treating chronic migraines, as it primarily focuses on symptom management rather than addressing the root causes such as fibrotic tissue, fascial restrictions, and underlying hormonal and nutritional imbalances. Without a comprehensive, holistic approach, the body remains stuck in this repetitive pattern, preventing true recovery.

Behavior Modification

Behavior modification is a therapeutic approach used to replace undesirable behaviors with more desirable ones through the systematic application of learning principles and techniques. It is rooted in the theories of operant conditioning developed by John B. Watson and B.F. Skinner. The fundamental premise is that behaviors can be learned and unlearned based on the consequences they produce.

Behavior modification can be an effective strategy for managing migraines by addressing lifestyle habits, environmental factors, and stressors that contribute to migraine frequency and severity. Many migraine triggers, such as poor sleep patterns, stress responses, dietary choices, and postural habits, develop over time. By using systematic techniques, individuals can adopt healthier behaviors that may reduce the intensity and frequency of migraines.

Identifying the Behaviors

The first step in behavior modification is identifying and clearly defining the behaviors that contribute to migraines. These may include:

- **Poor Sleep Hygiene:** Inconsistent sleep schedules, excessive screen time before bed, or inadequate sleep duration.
- **Stress-Induced Habits:** Engaging in negative coping mechanisms such as excessive caffeine consumption, lack of relaxation practices, or overcommitment to responsibilities.
- **Dietary Triggers:** Consuming foods known to trigger migraines, such as processed meats, caffeine, alcohol, or artificial sweeteners.
- **Postural Issues:** Forward head posture, prolonged screen use, or improper workplace ergonomics, which can lead to muscular tension and migraine onset.

Setting Goals

Setting **SMART goals** (Specific, Measurable, Achievable, Relevant, and Time-bound) helps individuals modify behaviors effectively. Examples include:

- **Improve sleep hygiene** by going to bed and waking up at the same time every day for four weeks.

- **Reduce stress-related behaviors** by practicing deep breathing exercises for five minutes, three times daily.
- **Eliminate dietary triggers** by tracking migraine occurrences and systematically removing suspected trigger foods for four weeks.
- **Enhance posture awareness** by taking a two-minute break every 30 minutes to stretch and adjust posture during screen use.

Techniques for Behavior Modification

Several techniques can be employed to modify behaviors linked to migraines:
- **Education and Awareness:** Many individuals unknowingly engage in behaviors that trigger migraines. Learning about how certain habits contribute to migraines can empower individuals to make informed changes.
- **Self-Monitoring:** Tracking migraine patterns, daily habits, and triggers using a migraine journal or mobile app helps identify patterns and adjust behaviors accordingly.
- **Positive Reinforcement:** Rewarding positive behaviors encourages adherence to healthier habits. This could include self-rewards for maintaining a consistent sleep routine, successfully eliminating a dietary trigger, or completing stress-reducing activities.
- **Cueing and Prompting:** Using reminders, alarms, or apps to prompt behaviors like hydration, stretching, posture adjustments, or mindfulness exercises can reinforce positive habits.
- **Feedback:** Seeking feedback from a healthcare provider, migraine specialist, or support group can provide accountability and adjustments to behavior modification strategies.
- **Modeling:** Observing others successfully managing migraines through behavior modification techniques, such as relaxation exercises or ergonomic adjustments, can inspire individuals to implement similar strategies.

Maintenance and Generalization

Once new behaviors are learned, they need to be maintained and applied across different situations. This includes:
- **Consistent Practice:** Continuing stress management techniques, sleep hygiene, and dietary awareness even after symptoms improve.

- **Social Support:** Engaging family, friends, or coworkers to encourage and remind individuals about their migraine management strategies.
- **Environmental Adjustments:** Modifying the home and work environment to support behavioral changes, such as investing in ergonomic furniture, reducing blue light exposure before sleep, or meal-prepping migraine-friendly foods.

Through these steps, behavior modification can help individuals reduce migraine severity and frequency by addressing modifiable lifestyle factors.

Conclusion

Following the recommendations outlined in the posture and behavior modification chapters can provide guidance on necessary behavior changes. For individuals experiencing persistent migraines despite behavioral adjustments, consulting a healthcare provider trained in behavioral therapy and migraine management is advisable. A behavioral therapist or migraine specialist can assess lifestyle patterns, triggers, and body mechanics to develop personalized behavior modification strategies. Those with postural-related migraines may require ergonomic corrections and targeted exercises. By addressing underlying habits, individuals can take a proactive role in reducing migraine occurrence and improving their overall well-being.

Conclusion

Conclusion

Healing from migraines requires a comprehensive approach that goes beyond simply managing symptoms. Throughout this book, we have explored seven natural strategies that address the root causes of migraines, helping you break free from chronic pain and regain control over your health. By identifying migraine-triggering foods, balancing vitamins, minerals, and hormones, and correcting posture, you can support your body's natural healing process. Managing stress, addressing fibrotic tissue and fascial restrictions, and modifying harmful behaviors further enhance recovery and migraine prevention.

One of the most critical aspects of this journey is ensuring that your body has the proper nutritional foundation to transition from chronic inflammation to full recovery. Deficiencies in essential vitamins, minerals, and hormones can prevent the body from properly regulating inflammation, repairing tissues, and restoring neurological balance. Many individuals with migraines suffer from underlying deficiencies without realizing it, which can keep them trapped in a cycle of pain, fatigue, and recurring headaches. From my clinical experience, migraine patients typically suffer from at least **three to six vitamin and mineral deficiencies**. To optimize the healing process, it is essential to work with a clinical nutritionist who can assess nutritional, vitamin, and mineral balance through comprehensive lab testing. Identifying and correcting deficiencies will enhance the body's ability to recover and improve the effectiveness of the other strategies presented in this book.

Each of the seven elements discussed plays a significant role in reducing migraine frequency and severity. Addressing only one or two areas may provide partial relief, but achieving lasting improvement requires a multi-faceted approach. Identifying food triggers and eliminating inflammatory foods can reduce unnecessary stress on the body, helping to prevent migraines. Maintaining proper posture and addressing musculoskeletal imbalances can further relieve tension that contributes to migraine development. Managing stress is crucial, as chronic stress leads to hormonal imbalances and nervous system overactivity, both of which can worsen migraine symptoms. Treating fibrotic tissue and fascial restrictions can improve circulation, reduce nerve compression, and promote tissue healing, all of which support long-term pain reduction. Behavior modification is equally important in changing habits and reinforcing positive lifestyle adjustments that prevent migraines from recurring.

By approaching migraine treatment with a holistic and personalized strategy, individuals can achieve sustainable relief and improved overall well-being. **The process of healing takes time and commitment**, but with the right knowledge and support, it is possible to regain control over your health. Taking proactive steps to address nutritional imbalances, lifestyle factors, and structural issues can transform the way the body responds to pain and restore balance. Working closely with healthcare professionals and making informed choices based on your unique needs will set the foundation for long-term success. Through consistent application of these principles, you can move beyond managing migraines and toward a healthier, pain-free life.

Recommended Resources

How to Access Online Content
1. Open the camera app on your smartphone.
2. Point the camera at the barcode.
3. A notification will appear with a link. Tap the notification to open the link in your browser.

1. Posture and Body Mechanics Training Videos

2. Case Studies and Recorded Live Treatment Videos

3. <u>Limited Time Offer</u>: FREE 30-minute Health Coach Consultation

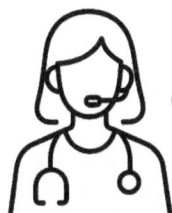

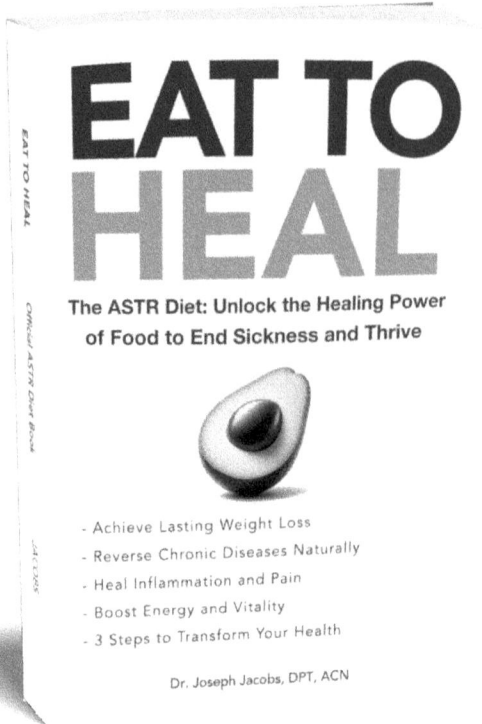

EAT TO
HEAL

The ASTR Diet: Unlock the Healing Power of Food to End Sickness and Thrive

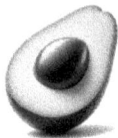

- Achieve Lasting Weight Loss
- Reverse Chronic Diseases Naturally
- Heal Inflammation and Pain
- Boost Energy and Vitality
- 3 Steps to Transform Your Health

Dr. Joseph Jacobs, DPT, ACN

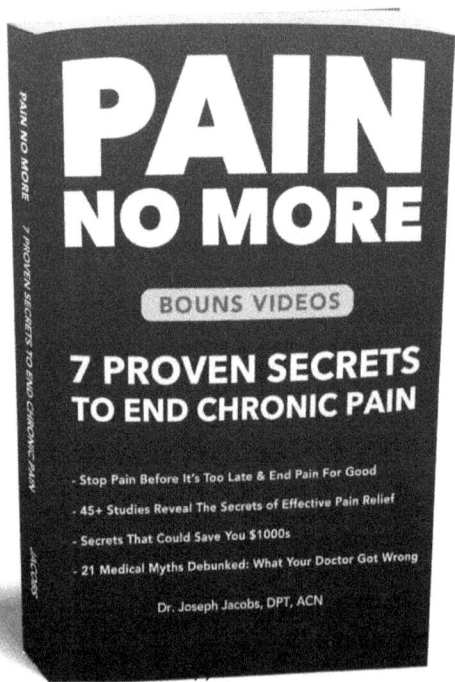

PAIN
NO MORE

BOUNS VIDEOS

7 PROVEN SECRETS
TO END CHRONIC PAIN

- Stop Pain Before It's Too Late & End Pain For Good
- 45+ Studies Reveal The Secrets of Effective Pain Relief
- Secrets That Could Save You $1000s
- 21 Medical Myths Debunked: What Your Doctor Got Wrong

Dr. Joseph Jacobs, DPT, ACN

BEATING
ANXIETY
&
DEPRESSION

BONUS VIDEOS

14 NATURAL SECRETS TO
A HAPPIER LIFE

- Conquer Anxiety & Depression Naturally
- Heal the Root Causes & Reclaim Your Life
- Created by a Doctor Who Conquered PTSD & Depression
- Science-Based Strategies for Lasting Change

Dr. Joseph Jacobs, DPT, ACN

REVERSING
DIABETES

10 NATURAL SECRETS TO REVERSE
DIABETES WITHOUT DRUGS

NORMAL

- Drug-Free, Side-Effect-Free, Science-Backed Healing
- Treat the Root Cause, Not Just the Symptoms
- Proven Natural Strategies That Get Results

Dr. Joseph Jacobs, DPT, ACN

REVERSING
HIGH BLOOD
PRESSURE

**7 NATURAL SECRETS TO SAFELY
LOWER BLOOD PRESSURE**

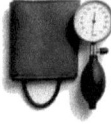

- Natural Solutions That Work
- Backed by Extensive Research
- Fix the Root Cause, Not Just the Numbers
- No Drugs, No Side Effects

Dr. Joseph Jacobs, DPT, ACN

BEATING
BACK PAIN

BONUS VIDEOS

7 NATURAL SECRETS FOR
LASTING RELIEF

- End Back Pain Naturally
- Clinically Tested, Doctor-Approved
- Fix the Root Causes, Not Just Symptoms
- Backed by Science & Research
- Created by a Doctor Who Beat Chronic Pain

Dr. Joseph Jacobs, DPT, ACN

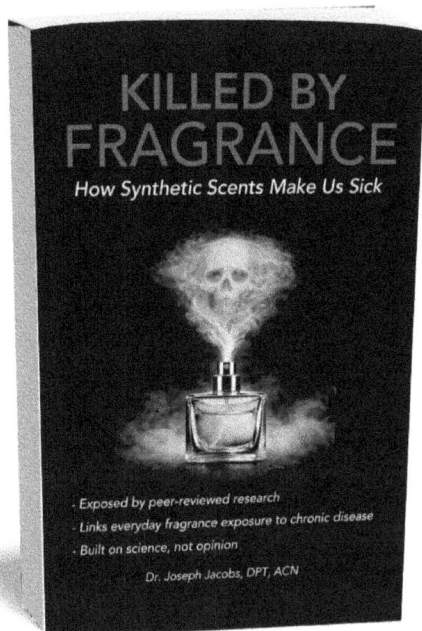

KILLED BY
FRAGRANCE
How Synthetic Scents Make Us Sick

- Exposed by peer-reviewed research
- Links everyday fragrance exposure to chronic disease
- Built on science, not opinion

Dr. Joseph Jacobs, DPT, ACN

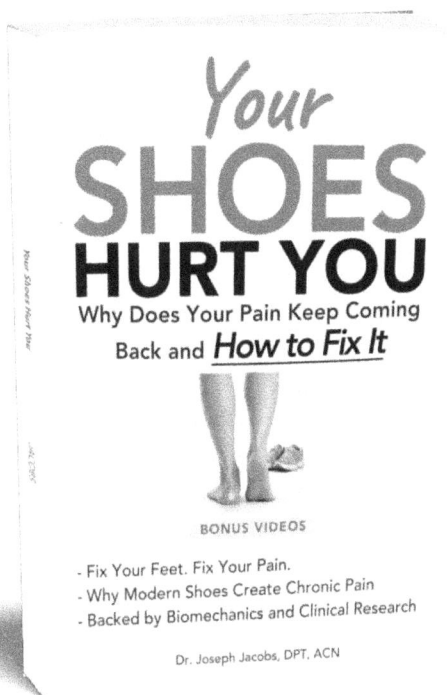

Your
SHOES
HURT YOU
Why Does Your Pain Keep Coming
Back and *How to Fix It*

BONUS VIDEOS

- Fix Your Feet. Fix Your Pain.
- Why Modern Shoes Create Chronic Pain
- Backed by Biomechanics and Clinical Research

Dr. Joseph Jacobs, DPT, ACN

Glossary

A
Acetylcholine – A neurotransmitter involved in nerve signal transmission, muscle movement, and cognitive function, which may play a role in migraine development.

Adrenal Fatigue – A condition where prolonged stress leads to dysregulated cortisol levels, potentially triggering migraines.

Amino Acids – The building blocks of proteins that play essential roles in neurotransmitter function, muscle repair, and brain health.

Antioxidants – Compounds that protect cells from oxidative stress, commonly found in fruits, vegetables, and certain supplements.

Artificial Sweeteners – Sugar substitutes like aspartame and sucralose that have been linked to migraines in sensitive individuals.

B
Beta-Blockers – A class of medications sometimes prescribed for migraine prevention due to their ability to regulate blood pressure and reduce vascular fluctuations.

Blood-Brain Barrier (BBB) – A protective barrier that controls substances entering the brain; dysfunction in this barrier has been linked to migraine pathophysiology.

Brainstem Dysfunction – Abnormal activity in the brainstem that may contribute to migraine development, particularly in regulating pain and sensory processing.

C
Circadian Rhythm – The body's natural sleep-wake cycle, which, when disrupted, can trigger migraines.

Cluster Headaches – Severe headaches often mistaken for migraines, characterized by intense pain around one eye and occurring in cyclical patterns.

Craniosacral Therapy – A hands-on therapy that uses gentle manipulation of the skull and spine to relieve tension and improve nervous system function.

D
Detoxification – The process of eliminating toxins from the body, which may help reduce inflammation and migraine frequency.

Dietary Histamine – A naturally occurring compound in certain foods (such as aged cheese and wine) that can trigger migraines in sensitive individuals.

Dopamine Dysregulation – An imbalance in dopamine, a neurotransmitter involved in mood and pain processing, which has been implicated in migraines.

E
Electrolyte Imbalance – A disruption in minerals such as sodium, potassium, and magnesium that can affect nerve function and contribute to migraines.

Elimination Diet – A structured approach to identifying food triggers by removing and gradually reintroducing specific foods.

Episodic Migraine – A form of migraine occurring fewer than 15 days per month, as opposed to chronic migraines.

F
Functional Medicine – A holistic healthcare approach that identifies and treats the root causes of disease rather than just managing symptoms.

Folate Deficiency – A lack of vitamin B9, which can contribute to migraine development and neurological dysfunction.

Food Sensitivities – Adverse reactions to specific foods, which may trigger migraines through inflammatory or immune responses.

G

Glossary

GABA (Gamma-Aminobutyric Acid) – A neurotransmitter that helps regulate nerve excitability; low levels are associated with increased migraine sensitivity.

Genetic Markers – Specific genes linked to an increased risk of migraines, such as those related to serotonin and vascular function.

Ginger – A natural anti-inflammatory herb that has been shown to reduce migraine symptoms in some studies.

H

HPA Axis (Hypothalamic-Pituitary-Adrenal Axis) – A system that regulates stress responses; dysfunction in this system can contribute to migraines.

Hyperalgesia – An increased sensitivity to pain, often seen in chronic migraine sufferers due to nervous system changes.

I

Inflammatory Cytokines – Proteins involved in immune responses that can contribute to neuroinflammation and migraine attacks.

Insulin Resistance – A metabolic condition where cells fail to respond effectively to insulin, potentially linking blood sugar fluctuations to migraines.

Intermittent Fasting – A dietary approach involving periods of eating and fasting, which may help reduce inflammation and improve metabolic health.

J

Jaw Misalignment (TMJ Dysfunction) – A condition where temporomandibular joint dysfunction contributes to tension headaches and migraines.

K

Keto Diet (Ketogenic Diet) – A low-carb, high-fat diet that some migraine sufferers use to stabilize blood sugar and reduce attacks.

Ketones – Alternative energy molecules produced when carbohydrate intake is low; some research suggests they may benefit migraine sufferers.

L

Lactic Acid Buildup – A condition resulting from metabolic stress, which can contribute to muscle tension and migraine symptoms.

Leaky Gut Syndrome – A digestive issue where the gut lining becomes permeable, allowing toxins to enter the bloodstream and potentially trigger migraines.

L-Theanine – An amino acid found in tea that promotes relaxation and may help with migraine-related stress.

M

Magnesium Deficiency – A common nutritional deficiency associated with increased migraine frequency and severity.

Mast Cell Activation – A condition where immune cells release excessive histamine, potentially triggering migraines.

Melatonin – A hormone that regulates sleep cycles; low levels are linked to migraine occurrence.

N

Nerve Compression – A condition where pinched nerves in the neck or spine contribute to migraine symptoms.

Neuropathic Pain – Pain caused by nerve dysfunction, which can be a factor in chronic migraines.

O

Omega-3 Fatty Acids – Anti-inflammatory fats found in fish and flaxseeds that may help reduce migraine severity.

Overuse Headache – A condition where excessive reliance on pain medications leads to rebound headaches.

Glossary

P

Postural Imbalance – Misalignment of the spine and neck that can increase muscle tension and trigger migraines.

Proprioception – The body's ability to sense its position in space, which can be affected by migraines.

R

Reactive Hypoglycemia – A condition where blood sugar drops suddenly after eating, which can trigger migraines.

Restorative Sleep – Deep sleep cycles that are essential for brain recovery and migraine prevention.

S

Sleep Apnea – A condition where breathing repeatedly stops during sleep, contributing to poor oxygen flow and increased migraine risk.

Spinal Alignment – The proper positioning of the spine, which plays a role in preventing tension-related migraines.

Stress Hormones – Hormones such as cortisol and adrenaline that, when imbalanced, can contribute to migraine onset.

T

Tryptophan – An amino acid precursor to serotonin, which helps regulate mood and migraine activity.

Trigger Points – Sensitive areas in muscles that can contribute to referred pain and migraine symptoms.

Tyramine – A compound found in aged foods (such as cheese and cured meats) that has been linked to migraines.

V

Vagus Nerve Stimulation (VNS) – A therapy that involves stimulating the vagus nerve to help manage migraines and neurological conditions.

Vestibular Migraine – A type of migraine associated with dizziness, balance issues, and vertigo.

Z

Zinc Deficiency – A nutritional deficiency that may contribute to immune dysfunction and increased migraine susceptibility.

References

1. Joseph J, Madison S, Tiffany J, Henry H, Mario V, et al . Evaluating the Effectiveness of Treatment Options for Pain: Literature Review.Ortho Res Online J. 3(5). OPROJ.000574.2018. DOI: 10.31031/OPROJ.2018.03.000574

2. University of Rochester Medical Center. (n.d.). The Biopsychosocial Approach. Retrieved from https://www.urmc.rochester.edu/medialibraries/urmcmedia/education/md/documents/biopsychosocial-model-approach.pdfhttps://www.cdc.gov/nchs/fastats/diseases-and-conditions.htm

3. Yaribeygi, H., Panahi, Y., Sahraei, H., Johnston, T. P., & Sahebkar, A. (2017). The impact of stress on body function: A review. EXCLI journal, 16, 1057-1072.https://www.merriam-webster.com/dictionary/disease

4. Engel GL: The need for a new medical model: a challenge for biomedicine. Science 1977;196:129-136.

5. Engel GL: The clinical application of the biopsychosocial model. Am J Psychiatry 1980;137:535-544. https://pubmed.ncbi.nlm.nih.gov/847460/

6. Frankel RM, Quill TE, McDaniel SH (Eds.): The Biopsychosocial Approach: Past, Present, Future.University of Rochester Press, Rochester, NY, 2003.

7. Borrell-Carrió F, Suchman AL, Epstein RM: The biopsychosocial model 25 years later: principles, practice, and scientific inquiry. Ann Fam Med 2004;2:576-582.

8. Cohen J, Brown Clark S: John Romano and George Engel: Their Lives and Work.University of Rochester Press, Rochester, NY, and Boydell and Brewer Limited, Suffolk UK, 2010.

9. Challenging Traditional Perspectives on Pain Relief | Dr. Jacobs TEDx Talk

10. Hannah K. Scott, Ankit Jain, Mark Cogburn: Behavior Modification. Treasure Island (FL): StatPearls Publishing; 2024 Jan. 2023 Jul 10.https://pubmed.ncbi.nlm.nih.gov/29083709/

11. Straube, S., Andrew Moore, R., Derry, S., & McQuay, H. J. (2010). Vitamin D and chronic pain. Pain, 149(1), 14-19. https://www.ncbi.nlm.nih.gov/pmc/articles/PMC4427945/

12. https://www.betterhealth.vic.gov.au/health/healthyliving/Vitamins-and-minerals

13. Tzenalis A, Beneka A, Malliou P, Godolias, G, Staurou N. The biopsychosocial treatment approach for chronic neck and back pain: A systematic review of randomized controlled trials. European Psychomotricity Journal. 2016; 8: 29-48.

14. Beardsley C, Škarabot J. Effects of self-myofascial release: A systematic review. Journal of Bodywork and Movement Therapies. 2015;19(4):747-758. doi:10.1016/j.jbmt.2015.08.007.

15. Reuben DB, Alvanzo AA, Ashikaga T, et al. National Institutes of Health Pathways to Prevention Workshop: The Role of Opioids in the Treatment of Chronic Pain. Annals of Internal Medicine. 2015;162(4):295-300. doi:10.7326/m14-2775.

16. ASAM Opioid Addiction 2016 Facts & Figures. American Society of Addiction Medicine

17. Prescription opioids and heroin epidemic in Georgia. Substance Abuse Research Alliance (SARA) | Georgia Prevention Project. 2017.

18. Bervoets DC, Luijsterburg PA, Alessie JJ, Buijs MJ, Verhagen AP. Massage therapy has short-term benefits for people with common musculoskeletal disorders compared to no treatment: a systematic review. Journal of Physiotherapy. 2015;61(3):106-116. doi:10.1016/j.jphys.2015.05.018.

19. Chou R, Deyo R, Friedly J, et al. Nonpharmacologic Therapies for Low Back Pain. Annals of Internal Medicine. 2017;167(8):493-505. doi:10.7326/I17-0395.

20. Miller J, Gross A, Dsylva J, et al. Manual therapy and exercise for neck pain: A systematic review. Manual Therapy. 2010;15(4):334-354. doi:10.1016/j.math.2010.02.007.

21. Cheatham SW, Lee M, Cain M, et al. : The efficacy of instrument assisted soft tissue mobilization: a systematic review. J Can Chiropr Assoc, 2016, 60: 200–211.

References

22. ngel G. The need for a new medical model: a challenge for biomedicine. Science. 1977;196(4286):129-136. doi:10.1126/science.847460.
23. Shete K, Suryawanshi P, Gandhi N. Management of low back pain in computer users: A multidisciplinary approach. Journal of Craniovertebral Junction and Spine. 2012;3(1):7-10. doi:10.4103/0974-8237.110117.
24. Kamper SJ, Apeldoorn AT, Chiarotto A, et al. Multidisciplinary biopsychosocial rehabilitation for chronic low back pain: Cochrane systematic review and meta-analysis. Bmj. 2015;350. doi:10.1136/bmj.h444.
25. Guzmán J, Esmail R, Karjalainen K, Malmivaara A Irvin E, Bombardier C et al. Multidisciplinary rehabilitation for chronic low back pain: systematic review BMJ 2001; 322 :1511-1516. doi:10.1136/bmj.322.7301.1511.
26. Korff MRV. Long-term use of opioids for complex chronic pain. Best Practice & Research Clinical Rheumatology. 2013;27(5):663-672. doi:10.1016/j.berh.2013.09.011.
27. Machado GC, Maher CG, Ferreira PH, Day RO, Pinheiro MB, Ferreira ML. Non-steroidal anti-inflammatory drugs for spinal pain: a systematic review and meta-analysis. Annals of the Rheumatic Diseases. 2017;76(7):1269-1278. doi:10.1136/annrheumdis-2016-210597.
28. Varas-Lorenzo C, Riera-Guardia N, Calingaert B, et al. Stroke risk and NSAIDs: a systematic review of observational studies. Pharmacoepidemiology and Drug Safety. 2011;20(12):1225-1236. doi:10.1002/pds.2227.
29. Turk DC, Okifuji A. Treatment of Chronic Pain Patients: Clinical Outcomes, Cost-Effectiveness, and Cost-Benefits of Multidisciplinary Pain Centers. Critical Reviews in Physical and Rehabilitation Medicine. 1998;10(2):181-208. doi:10.1615/critrevphysrehabilmed.v10.i2.40.
30. Mavrocordatos et al. Benefits of the multidisciplinary team for the patient
31. Espejo-Antúnez L, Tejeda JF-H, Albornoz-Cabello M, et al. Dry needling in the management of myofascial trigger points: A systematic review of randomized controlled trials. Complementary Therapies in Medicine. 2017;33:46-57. doi:10.1016/j.ctim.2017.06.003.
32. Jacobs J, Wilson J, Ireland K. Advanced Soft Tissue Release® (ASTR®) Long- and Short-Term Treatment Results for Patients with Neck Pain. MOJ Orthopedics & Rheumatology. 2016;5(4). doi:10.15406/mojor.2016.05.00188.
33. Yuan Q, Wang P, Liu L, et al. Acupuncture for musculoskeletal pain: A meta-analysis and meta-regression of sham-controlled randomized clinical trials. Scientific Reports. 2016;6:30675. doi:10.1038/srep30675.
34. Madsen MV, Gotzsche PC, Hrobjartsson A. Acupuncture treatment for pain: systematic review of randomised clinical trials with acupuncture, placebo acupuncture, and no acupuncture groups. Bmj. 2009;338. doi:10.1136/bmj.a3115.
35. Furlan, Andrea. Systematic review of acupuncture for chronic low-back pain . Japanese Acupuncture and Moxibustion, 2010; .6(1): 37-44
36. Rubinstein SM, Terwee CB, Assendelft WJ, Boer MRD, Tulder MWV. Spinal manipulative therapy for acute low-back pain. Spine. 2011;36(13):825-846. doi:10.1002/14651858.cd008880.pub2.
37. Gattie E, Cleland JA, Snodgrass S. The Effectiveness of Trigger Point Dry Needling for Musculoskeletal Conditions by Physical Therapists: A Systematic Review and Meta-analysis. Journal of Orthopaedic & Sports Physical Therapy. 2017;47(3):133-149. doi:10.2519/jospt.2017.7096.
38. Dunning J, Butts R, Mourad F, Young I, Flannagan S, Perreault T. Dry needling: a literature review with implications for clinical practice guidelines. Physical Therapy Reviews. 2014;19(4):252-265. doi:10.1179/1743288x13y.0000000118.
39. Morihisa R Eskew J McNamara A, et al. Dry Needling in subject with muscular trigger points in the lower quarter: a systematic review. Int J Sports Phys Ther. 2016;11(1):1-14.

40. Cotchett MP, Landorf KB, Munteanu SE. Effectiveness of dry needling and injections of myofascial trigger points associated with plantar heel pain: a systematic review. J Foot Ankle Res. 2010;3:18.

41. Cummings TM, White AR. Needling therapies in the management of myofascial trigger point pain: a systematic review.Arch Phys Med Rehabil 2001;82:986-92.

42. Xue CC, Helme RD, Gibson S, et al. Effect of electroacupuncture on opioid consumption in patients with chronic musculoskeletal pain: protocol of a randomised controlled trial. Trials. 2012;13:169. doi:10.1186/1745-6215-13-169.

43. Scott N. A., Guo B., Barton P. M., Gerwin R. D. Trigger point injections for chronic non-malignant musculoskeletal pain: a systematic review. Pain Medicine. 2009;10(1):54–69. doi: 10.1111/j.1526-4637.2008.00526.x.

44. Ernst E, Canter PH. A systematic review of systematic reviews of spinal manipulation. Journal of the Royal Society of Medicine. 2006;99(4):192-196.

45. Young JL, Walker D, Snyder S, Daly K. Thoracic manipulation versus mobilization in patients with mechanical neck pain: a systematic review. J Man Manip Ther. 2014;22:141–153. doi: 10.1179/2042618613Y.0000000043.

46. Filho JCANDS, Gurgel JL, Porto F. Effects of stretching exercises for posture correction: systematic review. Manual Therapy, Posturology & Rehabilitation Journal. 2014;12:200. doi:10.17784/mtprehabjournal.2014.12.200.

47. Thacker SB, Gilchrist J, Stroup DF, Kimsey CD. The Impact of Stretching on Sports Injury Risk: A Systematic Review of the   Literature. Medicine & Science in Sports & Exercise. 2004;36(3):371-378. doi:10.1249/01.mss.0000117134.83018.f7.

48. Small K, Naughton LM, Matthews M. A Systematic Review into the Efficacy of Static Stretching as Part of a Warm-Up for the Prevention of Exercise-Related Injury. Research in Sports Medicine. 2008;16(3):213-231. doi:10.1080/15438620802310784.

49. Borchers et al. A Systematic Review of the Effectiveness of Kinesis Taping for Musculoskeletal Injury

50. Gordon R, Bloxham S. A Systematic Review of the Effects of Exercise and Physical Activity on Non-Specific Chronic Low Back Pain. Healthcare. 2016;4(2):22. doi:10.3390/healthcare4020022.

51. Ajimsha M, Al-Mudahka NR, Al-Madzhar J. Effectiveness of myofascial release: Systematic review of randomized controlled trials. Journal of Bodywork and Movement Therapies. 2015;19(1):102-112. doi:10.1016/j.jbmt.2014.06.001.

52. Desmeules et al. Impingement Syndrome: also called Swimmer's Shoulder

53. Desmeules FCA, Côté CH, Frémont P. Therapeutic Exercise and Orthopedic Manual Therapy for Impingement Syndrome: A Systematic Review. Clinical Journal of Sport Medicine. 2003;13(3):176-182. doi:10.1097/00042752-200305000-00009.

54. Gross A, Kay TM, Paquin J-P, et al. Exercises for mechanical neck disorders. Cochrane Database of Systematic Reviews. 2015. doi:10.1002/14651858.cd004250.pub5.

55. Saragiotto BT, Maher CG, Yamato TP, et al. Motor control exercise for chronic non-specific low-back pain. Cochrane Database of Systematic Reviews. August 2016. doi:10.1002/14651858.cd012004.

56. Cheatham SW, Kolber MJ, Cain M, et al. The Effects of Self-Myofascial Release Using a Foam Roll or Roller Massager on Joint Range of motion, muscle recovery, and performance: A Systematic Review. International Journal of Sport Physical Therapy. 2015 Nov;10(6):827-38.

57. Castro-Sánchez AMCAD, Matarán-Peñarrocha GA, Arroyo-Morales M, Saavedra-Hernández M, Fernández-Sola C, Moreno-Lorenzo C. Effects of myofascial release techniques on pain, physical function, and postural stability in patients with fibromyalgia: a randomized controlled trial. Clinical Rehabilitation. 2011;25(9):800-813. doi:10.1177/0269215511399476.

58. Furlan A, Yazdi F. Complementary and Alternative Therapies for Back Pain II.

59. Penas C, Campo M. Manual therapies in myofascial trigger point treatment: a systematic review. Journal of Bodywork and Movement Therapies. January 2005.

60. Vernon H, Schneider M. Chiropractic Management of Myofascial Trigger Points and Myofascial Pain Syndrome: A Systematic Review of the Literature. Journal of Manipulative and Physiological Therapeutics Vol 32 Iss 1. January 2009.

61. Kim JH, Lee HS, Park SW. Effects of the active release technique on pain and range of motion of patients with chronic neck pain. Journal of Physical Therapy Science. 2015;27(8):2461-2464. doi:10.1589/jpts.27.2461.

62. Wong CK, Abraham T, Karimi P, Ow-Wing C. Strain counterstrain technique to decrease tender point palpation pain compared to control conditions: a systematic review with meta analysis. Journal of Bodywork and Movement Therapies. 2014 Apr;18(2):16573. doi: 10.1016/j.jbmt.2013.09.010.

63. Jakel A, Von Hauenschild P. A systematic review to evaluate the clinical benefits of craniosacral therapy. Complementary Therapies in Medicine. 2012 Dec;20(6):45665. doi: 10.1016/j.ctim.2012.07.009.

64. Green C, Martin CW, Bassett K, Kazanjian A. A systematic review of craniosacral therapy: biological plausibility, assessment reliability and clinical effectiveness. Complementary Therapies in Medicine. 1999. 7, 201-207

65. Clare A Helen, Adams Roger, Maher G Christoper. A systematic review of efficacy of McKenzie therapy for spinal pain. Australian Journal of Physiotherapy. 2004 Vol. 50.

66. Machado, Luciana Andrade Carneiro; de Souza, Marcelo von Sperling ; Ferreira, Paulo Henrique ; Ferreira, Manuela Loureiro. The McKenzie Method for Low Back Pain: A Systematic Review of the Literature with a Meta-Analysis Approach. April 20th, 2006. Volume 31 - Issue 9 - p E254-E262 doi: 10.1097/01.brs.0000214884.18502.93

67. Ravenek, M. J., Hughes, I. D., Ivanovich, N., Tyrer, K., Desrochers, C., Klinger, L., & Shaw, L. (2010). A systematic review of multidisciplinary outcomes in the management of chronic low back pain. IOS Press. Retrieved from http://web.a.ebscohost.com.vanguard.idm.oclc.org/ehost/pdfviewer/pdfviewer?vid=12&sid=06eb7fdd-c09c-407c-8fae-c12356183f73%40sessionmgr4010.

68. Kaija A Karjalainen MD. Multidisciplinary Biopsychosocial Rehabilitation for Subacute Low Back Pain in Working-Age Adults: A Systematic Review Within the Framework of the Cochrane Collaboration Back Review Group http://journals.lww.com/spinejournal/Abstract/2001/02010/Multidisciplinary_Biopsychosocial_Rehabilitation.11.aspx

69. Maria Ospina, Christa Harstall. Multidisciplinary Pain Programs for Chronic Pain: Evidence from Systematic Reviews. https://www.researchgate.net/publication/237306550_Multidisciplinary_Pain_Programs_for_Chronic_Pain_Evidence_from_Systematic_Reviews

70. Van Geen et al. The Long-term Effect of Multidisciplinary Back Training: A Systematic Review. http://journals.lww.com/spinejournal/Abstract/2007/01150/The_Long_term_Effect_of_Multidisciplinary_Back.17.aspx

71. Wynn, T. A. (2012). Mechanisms of fibrosis: therapeutic translation for fibrotic disease. Nature medicine, 18(7), 1028-1040.

72. Occupational Safety and Health Administration. (n.d.). Computer Workstations eTool: Proper Position. Retrieved from http://www.osha.gov/SLTC/etools/computerworkstations/positions.html[1]

References

73. Dahlhamer, J. (n.d.). Prevalence of chronic pain and high-impact chronic pain among adults in the U.S. Retrieved from https://consensus.app/papers/prevalence-chronic-pain-highimpact-chronic-pain-among-dahlhamer/

74. Johannes, C. B. (2018). Prevalence of Pain in United States Adults: Results from the Johannes Study. Retrieved from https://consensus.app/papers/prevalence-pain-united-states-adults-results-johannes/

75. Vos, T., Lim, S. S., Abbafati, C., Abbas, K. M., Abbasi, M., Abbasifard, M., ... & Murray, C. J. L. (2018). Global, regional, and national incidence, prevalence, and years lived with disability for 354 diseases and injuries for 195 countries and territories, 1990–2017: a systematic analysis for the Global Burden of Disease Study 2017. The Lancet, 392(10159), 1789-1858. https://doi.org/10.1016/S0140-6736(18)32279-7

76. Hay, S. I., Abajobir, A. A., Abate, K. H., Abbafati, C., Abbas, K. M., Abd-Allah, F., ... & Murray, C. J. L. (2018). Global, regional, and national disability-adjusted life-years (DALYs) for 333 diseases and injuries and healthy life expectancy (HALE) for 195 countries and territories, 1990–2016: a systematic analysis for the Global Burden of Disease Study 2016. The Lancet, 390(10100), 1260-1344. https://doi.org/10.1016/S0140-6736(17)32130-X

77. Rock, K. L., Kono, H. (2008). The inflammatory response to cell death. Annual Review of Pathology: Mechanisms of Disease, 3, 99-126. https://doi.org/10.1146/annurev.pathmechdis.3.121806.151456

78. Hurley ET, Calvo-Munoz I, Desai N, Buckley PS, Tanji JL, Greenbaum BS, Feeley BT. Systematic Review and Meta-Analysis of Nonoperative Platelet-Rich Plasma Shoulder Injections for Rotator Cuff Pathology. Arthroscopy. 2021 Jan;37(1):265-278. doi: 10.1016/j.arthro.2020.08.035. Epub 2020 Sep 11. PMID: 33131197

79. Ebadi S, Henschke N, Forogh B, Ansari NN, van Tulder M, Bagheri R, Fallah E. Therapeutic Ultrasound for Chronic Pain Management in Joints: A Systematic Review. Pain Pract. 2020 Apr;20(4):425-442. doi: 10.1111/papr.12864. Epub 2019 Dec 16. PMID: 31095336.

80. Xu C, Michail M, Cheng L, Cheng L, Xie X, Zhang M. A systematic review of clinical studies on electrical stimulation therapy for patients with neurogenic bowel dysfunction after spinal cord injury. Spinal Cord. 2018 Nov;56(11):1059-1073. doi: 10.1038/s41393-018-0180-z. Epub 2018 Aug 10. PMID: 30313096

81. Arroll B, Goodyear-Smith F. Corticosteroid injections for osteoarthritis of the knee: meta-analysis. BMJ. 2004 Apr 10;328(7444):869. doi: 10.1136/bmj.38039.573970.7C. PMID: 15039276; PMCID: PMC387493.

82. Ekhtiari S, Horner NS, Hincapie CA, Aleem AW, Cheng J, Boettner F, Piuzzi NS. Intra-articular saline injection is as effective as corticosteroids, platelet-rich plasma and hyaluronic acid for hip osteoarthritis pain: a systematic review and network meta-analysis of randomised controlled trials. Br J Sports Med. 2021 Mar;55(5):256-263. doi: 10.1136/bjsports-2020-102195. Epub 2020 Aug 10. PMID: 32788249.

83. Conaghan PG, Kloppenburg M. Debate: Intra-articular steroid injections for osteoarthritis – harmful or helpful? Osteoarthritis and Cartilage Open. 2023 Mar;5:100218. doi: 10.1016/j.ocarto.2023.100218

84. Sousa Filho LF, Barbosa Santos MM, dos Santos GHF, Araújo AC, Jennings F, Calders P, Ferreira GE. Corticosteroid injection or dry needling for musculoskeletal pain and disability? A systematic review and GRADE evidence synthesis. Chiropr Man Therap. 2021 Dec 16;29(1):49. doi: 10.1186/s12998-021-00408-y. PMID: 34920524; PMCID: PMC8683524.

85. Coombes BK, Bisset L, Connelly LB, Brooks P, Vicenzino B. Optimising corticosteroid injection for lateral epicondylalgia with the addition of physiotherapy: A protocol for a randomised

References

control trial with placebo comparison. BMC Musculoskelet Disord. 2009 May 7;10:76. doi: 10.1186/1471-2474-10-76. PMID: 19422718; PMCID: PMC2688524.

86. Stecco, C. (2015). Functional Atlas of the Human Fascial System. Churchill Livingstone Elsevier.
87. Stecco, L. (2016). Atlas of Physiology of the Muscular Fascia. Piccin.
88. Bordoni, B., & Zanier, E. (2015). Understanding fibroblasts in order to comprehend the osteopathic treatment of the fascia. *Evidence-Based Complementary and Alternative Medicine, 2015*. https://doi.org/10.1155/2015/860934
89. Gauglitz, G., Korting, H., Pavicic, T., Ruzicka, T., & Jeschke, M. (2011). Hypertrophic scarring and keloids: Pathomechanisms and current and emerging treatment strategies. *Molecular Medicine, 17*(1-2), 113-125. https://doi.org/10.2119/molmed.2009.00153
90. McCulloch, J., & Kloth, L. (2010). Wound Healing: Evidence-Based Management (4th ed.).
91. Bordoni, B., & Zanier, E. (2015). Anatomic connections of the diaphragm: Influence of respiration on the body system. *Journal of Multidisciplinary Healthcare, 8*, 281-291. https://doi.org/10.2147/JMDH.S70111
92. Gauglitz, G. G., Korting, H. C., Pavicic, T., Ruzicka, T., & Jeschke, M. G. (2011). Hypertrophic scarring and keloids: Pathomechanisms and current and emerging treatment strategies. *Molecular Medicine, 17*(1-2), 113-125. https://doi.org/10.2119/molmed.2009.00153
93. Kumka, M., & Bonar, J. (2012). Fascia: A morphological description and classification system based on a literature review. *Journal of the Canadian Chiropractic Association, 56*(3).
94. Benjamin, M. (2009). The fascia of the limbs and back. *Journal of Anatomy, 214*. https://doi.org/10.1111/j.1469-7580.2008.01011.x
95. Barnes, J. (1990). *Myofascial Release*. Paoli, PA: John F. Barnes, P.T. and Rehabilitation Services, Inc.
96. Yang, C., Du, Y., Wu, J., et al. (2015). Fascia and Primo Vascular System. *Evidence-Based Complementary and Alternative Medicine, 2015*, 1-6. https://doi.org/10.1155/2015/303769
97. Findley, T. W. (2011). Fascia Research from a Clinician/Scientist's Perspective. *International Journal of Therapeutic Massage and Bodywork, 4*(4), 1-6.
98. Willard, F. H., Vleeming, A., Schuenke, M. D., Danneels, L., & Schleip, R. (2012). The thoracolumbar fascia: Anatomy, function and clinical considerations. *Journal of Anatomy, 221*, 507-536. https://doi.org/10.1111/j.1469-7580.2012.01511.x
99. Fallon, S. (2012). Nourishing Traditions: The Cookbook that Challenges Politically Correct Nutrition and the Diet Dictocrats.
100. Thompson, J. (4th ed.). Nutrition: An Applied Approach.
101. Wilson, J., & Lowery, R. (2017). The Ketogenic Bible: The Authoritative Guide to Ketosis.
102. Mercola, J. (2017). Fat for Fuel: A Revolutionary Diet to Combat Cancer, Boost Brain Power, and Increase Your Energy.
103. Litchford, M. (2012). Nutrition Focused Physical Assessment: Making Clinical Connections.
104. Vasquez, A. (Date not provided). Textbook of Clinical Nutrition and Functional Medicine, Vol. 1: Essential Knowledge for Safe Action and Effective Treatment (Inflammation Mastery & Functional Inflammology).
105. Bennett, P., & Bland, J. (2010). *Textbook of Functional Medicine*.
106. Sanchez A, Reeser JL, Lau HS, Yahiku PY, Willard RE, McMillan PJ, Cho SY, Magie AR, Register UD. Role of sugars in human neutrophilic phagocytosis. Am J Clin Nutr. 1973 Nov;26(11):1180-4. doi: 10.1093/ajcn/26.11.1180. PMID: 4541857.
107. IASTM Image: https://www.temu.com/5pcs-set-stainless-steel-iastm-therapy-massage-tools-tissue-fascia-recovery-muscle-massager-guasha-scraping-gua-sha-massage-tool-g-601099540868938.html?
108. Case Studies Video Link: https://advancedsofttissuerelease.com/treatment-videos-2/

References

109. Computer posture image source: https://www.osha.gov/etools/computer-workstations

110. Joseph J, Madison S, Tiffany J, Henry H, Mario V, et al . Evaluating the Effectiveness of Treatment Options for Pain: Literature Review.Ortho Res Online J. 3(5). OPROJ.000574.2018. DOI: 10.31031/OPROJ.2018.03.000574

111. University of Rochester Medical Center. (n.d.). The Biopsychosocial Approach. Retrieved from https://www.urmc.rochester.edu/medialibraries/urmcmedia/education/md/documents/biopsychosocial-model-approach.pdfhttps://www.cdc.gov/nchs/fastats/diseases-and-conditions.htm

112. Yaribeygi, H., Panahi, Y., Sahraei, H., Johnston, T. P., & Sahebkar, A. (2017). The impact of stress on body function: A review. EXCLI journal, 16, 1057-1072.https://www.merriam-webster.com/dictionary/disease

113. Chou R, Deyo R, Friedly J, et al. Nonpharmacologic Therapies for Low Back Pain. Annals of Internal Medicine. 2017;167(8):493-505. doi:10.7326/l17-0395.

114. Miller J, Gross A, Dsylva J, et al. Manual therapy and exercise for neck pain: A systematic review. Manual Therapy. 2010;15(4):334-354. doi:10.1016/j.math.2010.02.007.

115. Cheatham SW, Lee M, Cain M, et al. : The efficacy of instrument assisted soft tissue mobilization: a systematic review. J Can Chiropr Assoc, 2016, 60: 200–211.

116. ngel G. The need for a new medical model: a challenge for biomedicine. Science. 1977;196(4286):129-136. doi:10.1126/science.847460.

117. Shete K, Suryawanshi P, Gandhi N. Management of low back pain in computer users: A multidisciplinary approach. Journal of Craniovertebral Junction and Spine. 2012;3(1):7-10. doi:10.4103/0974-8237.110117.

118. Kamper SJ, Apeldoorn AT, Chiarotto A, et al. Multidisciplinary biopsychosocial rehabilitation for chronic low back pain: Cochrane systematic review and meta-analysis. Bmj. 2015;350. doi:10.1136/bmj.h444.

119. Guzmán J, Esmail R, Karjalainen K, Malmivaara A Irvin E, Bombardier C et al. Multidisciplinary rehabilitation for chronic low back pain: systematic review BMJ 2001; 322 :1511-1516. doi:10.1136/bmj.322.7301.1511.

120. Korff MRV. Long-term use of opioids for complex chronic pain. Best Practice & Research Clinical Rheumatology. 2013;27(5):663-672. doi:10.1016/j.berh.2013.09.011.

121. Machado GC, Maher CG, Ferreira PH, Day RO, Pinheiro MB, Ferreira ML. Non-steroidal anti-inflammatory drugs for spinal pain: a systematic review and meta-analysis. Annals of the Rheumatic Diseases. 2017;76(7):1269-1278. doi:10.1136/annrheumdis-2016-210597.

122. Varas-Lorenzo C, Riera-Guardia N, Calingaert B, et al. Stroke risk and NSAIDs: a systematic review of observational studies. Pharmacoepidemiology and Drug Safety. 2011;20(12):1225-1236. doi:10.1002/pds.2227.

123. Turk DC, Okifuji A. Treatment of Chronic Pain Patients: Clinical Outcomes, Cost-Effectiveness, and Cost-Benefits of Multidisciplinary Pain Centers. Critical Reviews in Physical and Rehabilitation Medicine. 1998;10(2):181-208. doi:10.1615/critrevphysrehabilmed.v10.i2.40.

124. Mavrocordatos et al. Benefits of the multidisciplinary team for the patient

125. Espejo-Antúnez L, Tejeda JF-H, Albornoz-Cabello M, et al. Dry needling in the management of myofascial trigger points: A systematic review of randomized controlled trials. Complementary Therapies in Medicine. 2017;33:46-57. doi:10.1016/j.ctim.2017.06.003.

126. Madsen MV, Gotzsche PC, Hrobjartsson A. Acupuncture treatment for pain: systematic review of randomised clinical trials with acupuncture, placebo acupuncture, and no acupuncture groups. Bmj. 2009;338. doi:10.1136/bmj.a3115.

127. Furlan, Andrea. Systematic review of acupuncture for chronic low-back pain . Japanese Acupuncture and Moxibustion, 2010; .6(1): 37-44

128. Rubinstein SM, Terwee CB, Assendelft WJ, Boer MRD, Tulder MWV. Spinal manipulative therapy for acute low-back pain. Spine. 2011;36(13):825-846. doi:10.1002/14651858.cd008880.pub2.

129. Stecco, C. (2015). Functional Atlas of the Human Fascial System. Churchill Livingstone Elsevier.

130. Stecco, L. (2016). Atlas of Physiology of the Muscular Fascia. Piccin.

131. Bordoni, B., & Zanier, E. (2015). Understanding fibroblasts in order to comprehend the osteopathic treatment of the fascia. *Evidence-Based Complementary and Alternative Medicine, 2015.* https://doi.org/10.1155/2015/860934

132. Gauglitz, G., Korting, H., Pavicic, T., Ruzicka, T., & Jeschke, M. (2011). Hypertrophic scarring and keloids: Pathomechanisms and current and emerging treatment strategies. *Molecular Medicine, 17*(1-2), 113-125. https://doi.org/10.2119/molmed.2009.00153

133. McCulloch, J., & Kloth, L. (2010). Wound Healing: Evidence-Based Management (4th ed.).

134. Bordoni, B., & Zanier, E. (2015). Anatomic connections of the diaphragm: Influence of respiration on the body system. *Journal of Multidisciplinary Healthcare, 8*, 281-291. https://doi.org/10.2147/JMDH.S70111

135. Gauglitz, G. G., Korting, H. C., Pavicic, T., Ruzicka, T., & Jeschke, M. G. (2011). Hypertrophic scarring and keloids: Pathomechanisms and current and emerging treatment strategies. *Molecular Medicine, 17*(1-2), 113-125. https://doi.org/10.2119/molmed.2009.00153

136. Kumka, M., & Bonar, J. (2012). Fascia: A morphological description and classification system based on a literature review. *Journal of the Canadian Chiropractic Association, 56*(3).

137. Benjamin, M. (2009). The fascia of the limbs and back. *Journal of Anatomy, 214.* https://doi.org/10.1111/j.1469-7580.2008.01011.x

138. Barnes, J. (1990). *Myofascial Release.* Paoli, PA: John F. Barnes, P.T. and Rehabilitation Services, Inc.

139. Yang, C., Du, Y., Wu, J., et al. (2015). Fascia and Primo Vascular System. *Evidence-Based Complementary and Alternative Medicine, 2015*, 1-6. https://doi.org/10.1155/2015/303769

140. Findley, T. W. (2011). Fascia Research from a Clinician/Scientist's Perspective. *International Journal of Therapeutic Massage and Bodywork, 4*(4), 1-6.

141. Willard, F. H., Vleeming, A., Schuenke, M. D., Danneels, L., & Schleip, R. (2012). The thoracolumbar fascia: Anatomy, function and clinical considerations. *Journal of Anatomy, 221*, 507-536. https://doi.org/10.1111/j.1469-7580.2012.01511.x

142. Litchford, M. (2012). Nutrition Focused Physical Assessment: Making Clinical Connections.

143. Vasquez, A. (Date not provided). Textbook of Clinical Nutrition and Functional Medicine, Vol. 1: Essential Knowledge for Safe Action and Effective Treatment (Inflammation Mastery & Functional Inflammology).

144. Bennett, P., & Bland, J. (2010). *Textbook of Functional Medicine.*

145. Sanchez A, Reeser JL, Lau HS, Yahiku PY, Willard RE, McMillan PJ, Cho SY, Magie AR, Register UD. Role of sugars in human neutrophilic phagocytosis. Am J Clin Nutr. 1973 Nov;26(11):1180-4. doi: 10.1093/ajcn/26.11.1180. PMID: 4541857.

146. IASTM Image: https://www.temu.com/5pcs-set-stainless-steel-iastm-therapy-massage-tools-tissue-fascia-recovery-muscle-massager-guasha-scraping-gua-sha-massage-tool-g-601099540868938.html?

147. Case Studies Video Link: https://advancedsofttissuerelease.com/treatment-videos-2/

148. Alpay, K., Ertas, M., Orhan, E. K., Ustay, D. K., Lieners, C., & Baykan, B. (2010). Diet restriction in migraine, based on IgG against foods: A clinical double-blind, randomised, cross-over trial. *Cephalalgia, 30*(7), 829–837.

References

149. Buettner, C., Nir, R. R., Bertisch, S. M., Bernstein, C., Schain, A., Mittleman, M. A., & Burstein, R. (2015). Simvastatin and vitamin D for migraine prevention: A randomized, controlled trial. *Annals of Neurology, 78*(6), 970–981.

150. Engel, G. L. (1977). The need for a new medical model: A challenge for biomedicine. *Science, 196*(4286), 129–136.

151. Fernández-de-Las-Peñas, C., Alonso-Blanco, C., Cuadrado, M. L., & Pareja, J. A. (2006). Forward head posture and neck mobility in chronic migraine. *The Journal of Headache and Pain, 7*(6), 372–379.

152. Goadsby, P. J., Holland, P. R., Martins-Oliveira, M., Hoffmann, J., Schankin, C., & Akerman, S. (2017). Pathophysiology of migraine: A disorder of sensory processing. *The Lancet Neurology, 16*(1), 25–38.

153. Gerwin, R. D. (2005). Myofascial pain syndrome: Mechanisms and management. *Journal of Musculoskeletal Pain, 13*(4), 3–11.
     MacGregor, E. A. (2014). Migraine in women. *Seminars in Neurology, 34*(5), 601–610.

154. Nestoriuc, Y., Rief, W., & Martin, A. (2008). Meta-analysis of biofeedback for migraine. *Pain, 138*(3), 504–515.

155. Penzien, D. B., Irby, M. B., Smitherman, T. A., Rains, J. C., & Houle, T. T. (2015). Behavioral interventions for migraine prevention. *Headache, 55*(1), 3–20.

156. Schoenen, J., Jacquy, J., & Lenaerts, M. (1998). Effectiveness of high-dose riboflavin in migraine prophylaxis. *Neurology, 50*(2), 466–470.

157. Stecco, C., Schleip, R., Klingler, W., et al. (2014). The role of fascia in musculoskeletal disorders. *Clinical Anatomy, 27*(2), 173–182.

158. Sun-Edelstein, C., & Mauskop, A. (2009). Role of magnesium in the pathogenesis and treatment of migraine. *Clinical Journal of Pain, 25*(5), 446–452.

Recommended Resources

How to Access Online Content
1. Open the camera app on your smartphone.
2. Point the camera at the barcode.
3. A notification will appear with a link. Tap the notification to open the link in your browser.

1. Posture and Body Mechanics Training Videos

2. Case Studies and Recorded Live Treatment Videos

3. <u>Limited Time Offer</u>: FREE 30-minute Health Coach Consultation

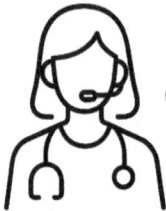